Also available from the
8 Keys to Mental Health Series

8 Keys to Mental Health Series
Babette Rothschild, Series Editor

The 8 Keys series of books provides readers with brief, inexpensive, and high-quality self-help books on a variety of topics in mental health. Each volume is written by an expert in the field, someone who is capable of presenting evidence-based information in a concise and clear way. These books stand out by offering consumers cutting-edge, relevant theory in easily digestible portions, written in an accessible style. The tone is respectful of the reader and the messages are immediately applicable. Filled with exercises and practical strategies, these books empower readers to help themselves.

8 KEYS TO MENTAL HEALTH THROUGH EXERCISE

CHRISTINA G. HIBBERT

FOREWORD BY BABETTE ROTHSCHILD

W.W. Norton & Company
Independent Publishers Since 1923
New York • London

Author's note: Certain names and identifying details of individuals whose case studies appear in these pages have been modified. A small number of individuals described are composites.

For information about permission to reproduce selections from this book, write to Permissions, W. W. Norton & Company, Inc., 500 Fifth Avenue, New York, NY 10110

For information about special discounts for bulk purchases, please contact W. W. Norton Special Sales at specialsales@wwnorton.com or 800-233-4830

Manufacturing by RR Donnelley Harrisonburg
Production manager: Christine Critelli

Library of Congress Cataloging-in-Publication Data

Names: Hibbert, Christina G., author.
Title: 8 keys to mental health through exercise / Christina G. Hibbert ; foreword by Babette Rothschild.
Other titles: Eight keys to mental health through exercise
Description: First edition. | New York : W.W. Norton & Company, [2016] | Includes bibliographical references and index.
Identifiers: LCCN 2015038856 | ISBN 9780393711226 (pbk.)
Subjects: LCSH: Mental illness—Alternative treatment. | Exercise therapy.
Classification: LCC RC480.5 .H46 2016 | DDC 616.89/1—dc23
LC record available at http://lccn.loc.gov/2015038856

W. W. Norton & Company, Inc.,
500 Fifth Avenue, New York, N.Y. 10110
www.wwnorton.com

W. W. Norton & Company Ltd.,
Castle House, 75/76 Wells Street, London W1T 3QT

1 2 3 4 5 6 7 8 9 0

To Braxton, Tre, Colton, Brody, Kennedy, & Sydney,
for inspiring me each day,
and for sometimes letting *me* inspire *you.*
You are my "why."

Contents

More Advance Acclaim for *8 Keys to Mental Health Through Exercise*

"I love this book because it combines solid research with practical, easy-to-follow steps to achieve the motivation and skills to exercise for better mental health. Being at your 'personal best' and, for parents, being a great role model to your children, means taking care of yourself first. If you're serious about getting fit mentally and physically, this book will help you to flourish!"

—**Dr. Rosina McAlpine**, parenting expert and author of *Inspired Children*; winwinparenting.com

"An incredible, accessible, and useful tool for ANYONE hoping to get exercising. Dr. Hibbert offers guidance, support, and tangible solutions to assist the reader through physical or mental roadblocks in order to strive to be their best self. I can't imagine anyone finishing the book without finding themself an improved individual. I'm grateful it has been written so that more people can benefit from exercise and tackle it through these carefully designed steps."

—**Dana Pieper**, creator of EveryBody Fitness

Foreword

Babette Rothschild, Series Editor

Everyone knows that exercise is good for our bodies and physical health. In addition to weight control, exercise improves and maintains overall health by supporting the immune system. Weight-bearing exercise keeps bones strong and aerobic exercise strengthens the heart and lungs. Really, the only negative thing about exercise is when people abuse it and *over*-exercise.

But did you know that exercise is also good for our *mental* health? In fact, it's so good for our minds that it is a near perfect adjunct (and in some cases, alternative) to psychotherapy. Study after study demonstrates that regular exercise improves mental health, as simply an antidote to a bad day or even to ease mild depression. It has also been shown to have a major positive impact on serious mental illnesses.

One of the best things about exercising for mental health is that anyone can do it, so long as they respect their individual circumstances. Someone who is housebound with agoraphobia can pace the living room, weight lift with water bottles, do sit-ups and push-ups on the floor, or even yoga. Someone in an office can do "desk workouts." People with physical limitations can find ways to exercise that work with their bodies. Many forms of exercise are free: walking, jogging, dancing in your living room, pick-up sports at the park with your friends, a myriad of exercise-with-me programs on television and online, and so on. Of course, if you want to spend money on classes, equipment, or a gym membership, all price ranges are available.

Perhaps best of all, exercise is accessible 24/7 – you can exercise whenever and (nearly) wherever you want. You can exercise alone or with companionship. You can make up your own program or utilize a trainer or consultant. The options and accessibility are literally endless. The only true barriers to exercise involve developing a program that suits your own level of fitness and personal preferences, and then…actually doing it.

Central to motivation is finding the right approach for you. *8 Keys to Mental Health Through Exercise* is designed to help you find your own unique way to exercise – which may or may not be like anyone else's. Everyone can utilize exercise to improve their mental health.

Whether you are an experienced and enthusiastic exerciser or a complete novice, this book has something to offer you. This book is more than just about exercise, it provides guidance in overcoming your personal roadblocks and in figuring out what approach to exercise is right for you.

Along the way you will learn about the most current research in psychology and neuroscience to help you understand how exercise benefits your body and mind. Mental disorders such as depression, anxiety, panic, bipolar disorder, and so on leave you feeling out of control of your mind and also sometimes out of control of your body because of the psychological and physical symptoms that accompany them. Engaging in individually tailored, personally planned and implemented exercise is a major way in which anyone can gain, regain, and restore a sense of self-control. Mastery over one's own body and mind has a powerfully positive effect on one's outlook and self-esteem.

This book will show you that the most simple as well as the most complex mental disorders respond extremely well to regular exercise. Hibbert will help you to identify, set, achieve, and maintain your individual, personal goals for exercise and mental health. Through the multitude of engaging examples from her own professional experience working with people who wanted to exercise for mental health, you will know that you are not alone, and that exercise can help you too.

In addition, Hibbert includes just the right amount of personal examples, so that she serves as a good role model but not a guru. Importantly, she recognizes that you will encounter roadblocks, that they are part of the process, progression *not* regression. She will help you to identify yours, and give you the tools to tackle and conquer them.

Each of us has our own unique challenges to engaging in, and sticking with, regular exercise. As a specialist in posttraumatic stress disorder (PTSD), and like most of my PTSD specialist colleagues, I have had my own trauma challenges to deal with throughout my life. A main symptom of my own PTSD has been persistent anxiety. A major exercise barrier for me was dealing with aerobic increases in respiration and heart rate that reminded me of states of anxiety and panic. This is common for people with PTSD as well as anxiety and panic disorder. Many years ago my own exercise program had to begin with *no* aerobic stimulation. I started instead by concentrating on slowly strengthening muscles. That was my personal in-road to being able to engage in exercise to improve my own mental health, including stabilization of my PTSD symptoms. Eventually, I was able to take up brisk walking and swimming, which I continue today. In fact, I am so convinced of the value of exercise in helping improve mental health that I devoted an entire chapter, "Get Moving," to this topic in my book *8 Keys to Safe Trauma Recovery.*

If you have any doubt about the intimate relationship between the mind and body you only have to look at the popular press to find a myriad of articles nearly every week espousing this important relationship: Nutrition and mood. Yoga and depression. Exercise and stress. Here is a little experiment about the connection between mind and body to get you started:

First check in with yourself and see what kind of mood you are in right now. How is your general outlook and mood? Then, in the chair you are sitting in reading this book, slump as much as you can. Really collapse your shoulders and duck your head toward your hips. If you do this correctly, your chest will be sunken-in, surrounded by your shoulders and head. Then pay attention to your mood. Has it changed? Do you feel better or worse than when you began this experiment? Many will feel some kind of dampening of mood in this posture. You may feel a little depressed or sad, less energetic or something like that. But we won't stop here.

Now, do the opposite: Sit up straight and tall. Gently bring your shoulders back a bit, not a military posture, more an attentive posture. Notice how when your chest opens up, your breathing becomes easier. Then notice your mood. Has it lightened any? Do you feel more positive or more energetic than in the slumping posture? Don't worry if you did not experience any differences, but most of you will now have a very tangible taste of the connection between mind and body: Slumping depresses mood, sitting up straight can lighten mood. Some people use this type of strategy to help them in challenging business situations. A colleague recently told me that before she has a meeting with her boss, she spends 5 minutes copying a Wonder Woman posture – a stance with arms raised and wrists crossed. She says it gives her a greater feeling of confidence and power when dealing with work challenges.

This book will give you the tools and confidence to make exercise your ally in mental health.

Hibbert will show you that there are ways to exercise that can compromise your mental health. Overdoing physical workouts can leave you feeling emotionally and physically wasted and like a failure. She also knows that engaging and sticking with exercise for mental health involves preparing the mind and emotions to be allies in the process. Do not worry that she will push you to bite off more than you can chew. In fact, she advocates for the opposite: starting with small steps, sometimes what seem to be ridiculously small. The idea is to begin with what you can do successfully, even if that is only a few steps. Building on small successes will lead to bigger successes and overall improved mental health. This book will help guide you to your right balance.

Acknowledgments

To my editor, Deborah Malmud, thank you for believing in me—for your encouragement, tough love, and patience. Without your foresight, insight, and sighting of my writing on exercise and mental health, I would never have been given the opportunity to create this book on this topic I love so dearly. I am deeply grateful.

To my husband, OJ, thank you for your endless support. Through the highs and lows of life (and writing), you're always there, offering encouraging words, pushing me forward, and bringing plenty of fun and laughter. You lighten me up! I truly could not do this without you.

To my children, to whom this book is dedicated—you are my motivation, and you definitely keep me moving! For exercising in the "dungeon" with me early in the mornings, for all the bike rides, jogs, arm wrestling, basketball games, and for out-performing me so quickly, motivating me to push myself even more. Being your mother is my greatest blessing. Now, if I could just keep pace with your flexibility, energy, and muscle "gains," I'd be set!

To Babette Rothschild, for your input and guidance as I fumbled toward creating this "8 Keys" book, I am grateful. Thank you for allowing me to be part of this series, and thank you for being my foreword author. None of this would be here without you.

To Elizabeth Baird, Alison Lewis, Benjamin Yarling, Angela Riley, Nate Cohan, my fabulous copyeditor, Elizabeth Shestak, and the entire team at Norton—for your tireless efforts on behalf of this book. You make me look good, and I am grateful!

Finally, to Mechelle, Tyler and Lindsay, Julie, Eric, Barb, and to all of the other individuals who allowed me to use their experiences with exercise for mental health in this book—I can't thank you enough. Through sharing our stories, we feel, we heal, we connect, and we grow. I am endlessly appreciative to have been able to grow in this project with you.

Introduction

Many years ago, a close friend confided she believed she was experiencing postpartum depression. This was her first baby, and she'd been dreaming of becoming a mom her whole life. Instead, she was met with sadness, anxiety, sleeplessness, and exhaustion. Only two months into being a mom, she felt completely hopeless.

Her husband tried to help, but didn't know what to do or say. They tried calling her doctor, but he just said, "Oh, it's probably the baby blues," and mailed her a pamphlet. This only made her more hopeless because her symptoms seemed like more than just the baby blues. They ended up moving in with her parents, sleeping on a mattress on their family room floor for three months, so her mom could help with the baby while my friend got some much-needed sleep and her poor husband continued to go to work and school.

Experiences like my friend's are common. An estimated 15% of women experience postpartum depression, and 10% experience depression in pregnancy (Postpartum Support International (PSI) 2015). New mothers may also experience pregnancy and postpartum anxiety, panic, obsessive-compulsive disorder, posttraumatic stress disorder, and even psychosis. It's not just women who might suffer following the birth of a child—an estimated 10% of fathers worldwide experience postpartum depression, too (Paulson & Bazemore, 2010). Together, perinatal mood and anxiety disorders have been called "the most common complication associated with childbirth" (PSI, 2015). And, as we see from the example above, mental illnesses like these can affect the entire family, causing stress and strain on important relationships and impacting everyday functioning.

This is just one of countless examples of everyday people living with various forms of mental illness, needing help, and not knowing where or how to find it. It's not just women in the childbearing years who might struggle; men and women of all ages, children, and teens are likewise affected by mental illness. It is a growing concern around the world.

Mental Illness: Prevalence, Treatment, and Barriers

According to the National Alliance on Mental Illness (NAMI, 2013):

- One in four American adults experience mental illness in any given year.
- One in seventeen adults live with a serious mental illness like major depression, bipolar disorder, or schizophrenia.
- 20% of teens, ages 13 to 18, and 13% of children ages 8 to 15, experience serious mental illness each year.
- 18.1% of Americans live with anxiety disorders, including generalized anxiety disorder, panic disorder, obsessive-compulsive disorder (OCD), posttraumatic stress disorder (PTSD), and phobias.
- 6.7% live with major depression, 2.6% live with bipolar disorder, and 1.1% live with schizophrenia.
- 9.2 million Americans have co-occurring addiction and mental illness.
- Depression and other mood disorders are the third most common cause of hospitalization for youth and adults ages 18 to 44 in the United States (NAMI, 2013).

And it's not just those in the United States who are suffering. Mental health disorders are common throughout the world, with a lifetime prevalence rate of 18.1% to 36.1%, according to a survey of 28 countries by the World Health Organization (Kessler et al., 2007. Most mental illness appears earlier in life, often in childhood or adolescence, and mental disorders are correlated with greater physical health problems down the road.

Unfortunately:

- An estimated 60% of American adults and almost half of children, ages 8 to 15, receive no treatment for their mental illness diagnoses.
- Minority populations with mental illness access treatment even less, with Hispanic and African Americans utilizing mental health services at approximately one-half the rate and Asian Americans at about one-third the rate of white populations, in a given year (NAMI, 2013).

In short, up to half of all mental disorders in the world remain untreated. This can lead to significant adverse consequences, including: poorer life choices and outcomes; increased risk of other disorders, both mental and physical; and great emotional and financial cost not only to those suffering, but to society as a whole (Kessler et al., 2007).

Adults suffering from serious mental illness die 25 years earlier than other Americans, on average, because they simply don't seek or receive treatment—treatment that is valid and could prolong life. That's the most tragic part—that the vast majority of mental illnesses are highly treatable, and yet most people still fail to seek treatment. The most common treatment methods include psychotropic medications, psychotherapy, social support/support groups, or a combination of these, which is considered the "gold standard" of care. Research shows that each of these treatment methods is effective in treating various mental health disorders, yet they still remain unutilized by such a large proportion of people. Why is this?

Why Mental Health Disorders Go Untreated

There are many reasons those suffering from mental illness may not seek treatment, but the following include those most common.

Stigma

Mental illness still carries a strong stigma, despite years of research explaining the biological, psychosocial, and environmental causes of mental illness. Mental health experts and advocates have worked tirelessly to ensure people understand that having a mental illness does not make one "weak" or "bad," yet many still feel they cannot, or had better not, for their own good, talk about their experiences with mental illness, fearing it will leave them marked by stigma. This prevents many from seeking help. As World Health Organization (WHO) researcher, Dr. T. Bedirhan Ustun, stated, "In every country there is a hidden or unhidden stigma. People are reluctant to admit that they have mental problems" (National Broadcasting Center News, 2004).

Medication also has a strong stigma. Many feel ashamed of taking psychotropic medications, even when those medications significantly help them become well. Therapy is similar, with many still feeling uncertain about sharing their personal lives with someone they've just met, no matter how qualified or beneficial that person's expertise. Simply reaching out for social support is often thwarted by the stigma of mental illness.

Side Effects of Medication

Though psychotropic medications, like antidepressants, have been proven highly effective in treating mental health disorders, most are typically associated with side effects—changes in appetite, sleep, or memory; dry mouth; drowsiness; headaches; or even sexual disturbance—that can be uncomfortable at best and exacerbate symptoms at worst (National Institute of Mental Health [NIMH], 2008). Together, the stigma of taking medication, combined with unwanted side effects, can lead many to resist medications or stop taking them after a short time, often cold turkey, which is contraindicated and may cause symptoms to flare up.

The Cost Involved

Finally, getting appropriate treatment for mental disorders comes at a significant cost—both financially and time-wise. For those without insurance, the costs required to establish the correct prescriptions, and then acquire those medications, can pose a huge financial burden. Even those with insurance often find their treatments of choice are not covered. Psychotherapy can also be a huge financial expense, with or without insurance, especially when therapists recommend weekly sessions.

There is also a significant time investment that goes into regular therapy sessions, psychiatric visits, or attending a support group. Many report they don't seek or follow through with treatment because they simply don't have the time. Though certainly the costs of *untreated* mental illness are far greater—financially, time-wise, and in overall life success and satisfaction—cost remains a barrier to treatment for many.

Can you relate to any of these barriers to treatment, either personally or through a loved one? Isn't it tragic to think so many people fail to seek and receive the support, care, and healing they need and deserve because of such things as stigma, side effects, and cost? This is especially tragic considering how effective the treatment methods can be.

There is far too much needless suffering in the world. Help and resources are available, but considering all these barriers, how can we ensure that people understand their resources, know where to turn for help, and actually get the help they need?

Exercise Overcomes Treatment Barriers

Enter exercise. Exercise is a valid and valuable treatment option, not only because it's been shown to improve a variety of mental disorders, but also because it overcomes these barriers to mental health treatment.

Stigma: unlike medication or therapy, there is no negative stigma associated with exercise. In fact, those who exercise are typically seen in a positive, healthy light by others and feel good about themselves for exercising. As we will see in the keys to come, exercise can improve self-confidence, self-esteem, and social wellness. Those suffering from mental disorders are likely to feel positively toward exercise as a treatment, which eliminates the stigma.

Side Effects: there are no known negative side effects of regular exercise, if done correctly, and that's what this book is here to teach. While exercise can certainly have some temporary negative side effects, like discomfort, muscle soreness, or shortness of breath, overall, the side effects of exercise are highly positive, as we will clearly outline in the keys to come. Also, exercise doesn't interact negatively with other treatments such as medication and therapy; it's actually considered a healthy addition to such treatment methods (Leith, 2009).

Cost: exercise is free. Beyond a good pair of shoes, running or walking requires no cost. Sure, some may join a fitness club, but it's not necessary in order to reap the mental health benefits of exercise. Additionally, while exercise does require a time commitment, as you will see in the coming keys, even 20 minutes, three times a week, can lead to improvements in mental health. Once we make exercise part of our daily routine, once we begin to experience the positive effects of it every day, the time it takes to exercise usually feels well worth it.

Exercise for Mental Health

Fortunately, my friend who was struggling with postpartum depression unintentionally stumbled upon exercise when she started taking long walks with the baby each day. Initially she just wanted to get out of the house and into the sun, but she soon started to feel how much exercise helped. "No, it didn't help," she said. "It saved me. It was one little thing I could do each day that lifted my mood. It let me feel like me again."

Exercise is one of the most powerful ways we can improve our mental health. I know, because I've studied the research and the research is definitive. I know, because I've worked with dozens of clients over the years, both as a psychologist, and before that as a certified fitness instructor, and I've witnessed the impact exercise has made in their lives. I know, because, I am the "friend" I wrote about above, and nineteen years later, exercise continues to be one of my main mental health supports. I hope that in reading 8 *Keys to Mental Health Through Exercise*, you will come to know and experience the mental health benefits of exercise, too.

What this Book is Not

This book is not a workout book

There are plenty of good books on how to get sculpted, toned, cut, trimmed, and pumped up. This isn't one of them. This book is about exercising—learning to move, becoming more physically active, and creating a habit of exercise that will provide mental and physical health benefits for life. While working out may become part of your exercise for mental health routine, the workouts themselves are not the main focus of this book.

This book is not a weight loss book

When most people think of exercise, their mind immediately goes to weight loss. This is not a weight loss book. It's a book about improving mental, and simultaneously, physical, health through exercise. It's a new way of viewing exercise—one that moves beyond physical appearance. Sure, some might experience weight loss as a side effect of exercise for mental health, but that's not our main goal in this book.

This book is not one you read casually and then put back on the shelf

This book is intended to make you think—about yourself, your thoughts, behaviors, habits, desires, drives, and motivations—and then, to do something with what you learn. I don't intend for you, the reader, to pick this book up, read it, and set it back down. I hope you choose to do the work as I lead you through the tools you need to build a habit of exercise for mental health, for life.

What this Book Is

This book is here to show you how to make exercise work for you

This book is about helping you overcome, become, and flourish in exercise and mental health. It's about teaching you the facts, skills, and tools you need to overcome your exercise roadblocks, become motivated, committed, and mentally stronger, and to flourish, reaping all the benefits exercise has to offer.

This book is set up in 8 Keys

In Part 1 (keys 1 through 3), you'll gain a deeper understanding and appreciation of all exercise has to offer. Key 1 provides a thorough look into the physical and mental health benefits of exercise, and then dives into common mental health issues and disorders, outlining how exercise is like medicine in treating them. Key 2 looks at the power of exercise on our self-esteem, confidence, and self-worth, and presents a new way to view and develop self-confidence and self-worth. Key 3 is about family—exercising as a family, that is—and how to make family exercise work for you.

In Part 2 (keys 4 through 6) we shift our focus to the mental preparation for exercise. Key 4 examines motivation and provides several theories and skills to help you become more motivated to exercise. Key 5 is all about how to change and strengthen your mind for exercise success, using strategies from cognitive-behavioral therapy (CBT) to teach specific tools needed to overcome excuses and build emotional and physical exercise stamina. Key 6 takes a deeper look into the most common roadblocks to exercise for mental health, and outlines a multitude of strategies for how to overcome them.

Finally, Part 3 (keys 7 and 8) describes how to implement and stick with an exercise for mental health program. Key 7 teaches the FITT principle, a simple method for establishing an effective exercise routine, and then shares specific strategies to help you tailor that program to your specific needs. Last but not least, Key 8 is about staying dedicated to exercise for mental health, showing you how to create your vision for lifelong wellness and make exercise a habit, while sharing principles of positive psychology to help you establish and achieve your long-term physical and mental health potential.

This book is designed to make you work—and grow

I've included a variety of activities designed to help you process and implement the principles presented in the book. My hope is that you'll take the time to answer the questions and complete the activities.

Each chapter contains three types of activities: "Reflection Questions," "Ponder This," and "Do This." "Reflection Questions" help you explore various aspects of yourself and then write about what you discover. "Ponder This" activities include ideas or concepts I'd like you to consider for a while, and "Do This" activities present specific actions I'm hoping you'll take.

As you do these short activities, you will gain a deeper understanding of your desires, needs, and roadblocks, as well as a stronger ability to apply the skills and tools you specifically need to your own life. They're here to make you work—to question, ponder, and hypothesize—but also help you synthesize and apply the new information in useful ways that help you grow. They are designed to help you personalize the contents of this book and make it work for you.

You may want to purchase a journal or notebook, or set up your computer, phone, or other device as a place to take notes. Keeping everything in one place is a great way to help you focus and get all you can out of this book.

This book is for everyone—beginners through experts

To those who are already avid exercisers, I say, read this book. I guarantee you will learn something new. This book will help you improve your mental health, gain more benefits from exercise, and facilitate you exercising your whole life long.

To those who are reading this and thinking, "I've never exercised before; I'm woefully out of shape or struggling with some pretty significant physical or mental health limitations," I say this book is especially for you. We will learn how to prepare your mind for exercise, as well as your body. We will walk through all you need to do to make exercise a permanent part of your life, and we will do this together—to help you reach your fullest mental and physical health potential.

And to everyone in between, I say, stick with me. You will soon understand what I mean when I say that exercise has the potential to not only improve your mental health, but to truly transform your life.

A Few More Important Things, Before We Begin

Since this book is about exercise, and mental health, there are a few things you need to remember:

1) *This book is not intended to replace medical or mental health care.* Though I hope it will be a valuable addition to your mental and physical health plan, this book is not a replacement for professional medical and mental health advice or treatment.

2) *Get doctor approval before beginning exercise.* Never begin a fitness program, even the one I will be outlining, without first getting your doctor's "okay." Especially if you're new to exercise, please visit your doctor, tell her of your intentions, and get her stamp of approval, and her guidance, before you begin. Even those who have been exercising for a while should seek advice from your doctor before significantly altering, adding to, or changing your exercise routine. Safety first. Always.

3) *Seek professional mental and physical health help as needed.* If you find that your mental health is in any way deteriorating, or if you face new mental or physical health challenges, I encourage you to seek help from a medical or mental health professional. Seeking help when we need it is one of the best ways to keep ourselves mentally, and physically, strong.

8 KEYS TO MENTAL HEALTH THROUGH EXERCISE

PART 1

Understand

KEY 1

HEAL YOUR MIND
AND BODY WITH EXERCISE

"It is exercise alone that supports the spirits, and keeps the mind in vigor."

—Marcus Cicero, 65 B.C.

You may have picked up this book because you have mental health concerns right now. You may have picked it up because you're considering exercise for the first time. You may have picked it up because you've been an avid exerciser but want to better understand the connection between exercise and mental health. Whatever your reasons, I'm grateful you've picked up this book, because exercise is one of the most powerful tools for improving not only your physical health, but also your mental and emotional health.

It appears that even Marcus Cicero knew this back in 65 B.C. Yet, it's taken centuries for the rest of us to fully understand the mental health benefits of exercise. Thanks to recent research and ever-expanding understanding of mental health issues and treatments, we now have the proof to back up what we long may have felt—that moving our body quite literally moves our mind.

The Mind-Body Connection

The mind and body are inextricably linked. This means that what happens to the mind affects the body, and vice versa. For example, if I live with untreated depression, my mental/emotional symptoms will eventually affect my physical health. Depression typically includes physical symptoms, like head/backaches, insomnia, and muscle tension or pain. Depression has also been shown to increase one's risk for disease and other conditions, like chronic pain or fatigue and even heart conditions. These disorders, in turn, can worsen depression. This is just one of many examples of how the mind and body are undeniably connected (Trivedi, 2004).

The mind-body connection has long been understood and used in healthcare by eastern cultures, and finally, the western world has also gotten on board, thanks to a boom in research over the years. The research is clear: our brain, immune and endocrine systems, nervous system, and the rest of our organs share a chemical language with our emotional responses. They are in continual communication with one another (Gordon, 2001). The mind and body are inseparable.

This means we can no longer afford to separate our mental well-being from our physical health care. The mind and body greatly influence and are influenced by one another and should be treated as such. It also means we must incorporate physical as well as mental/emotional treatments if we want to overcome emotional distress and mental illness. Simply put, if we want to be well, and to one day flourish—or, as I call it, to become "even better than better" (Hibbert, 2013, p. 401)—then we must respect the mind-body connection.

Exercise for Mental (and Physical) Health

Exercise is the perfect way to achieve and balance mental and physical health. Exercise strengthens our heart, muscles, and helps treat a variety of health conditions, while also strengthening emotional resilience, mental clarity, and treating mental illness.

Research shows there are just as many mental health benefits of exercise as there are physical, yet most adults (81.6%) and adolescents (81.8%) fail to get the recommended amount of daily exercise (United States Department of Health and Human Services [USD-HHS], 2008). Why are many not exercising when the benefits are so great? Most people don't understand the physical and mental health benefits of exercise, and most don't know how to make exercise work for them.

We'll discuss the "how's" of exercise in keys 4 through 8, but first, let's examine the research on the many physical, and especially mental, health benefits exercise has to offer.

The Physical Health Benefits of Exercise

The first research study confirming the physical health benefits of exercise wasn't conducted until 1949. This study, by epidemiologist Jerry Morris, compared bus drivers with the more active bus conductors and was the first to prove a link between a sedentary lifestyle and heart disease (Morris, 1958). Morris was consequently credited as "the man who invented exercise" (Kuper, 2009).

Today, we have a plethora of research demonstrating the physical health gains of exercise. Exercise is correlated with the following desirable health benefits:

- Weight loss and weight control—healthy weight loss is important not just for looking good. Losing weight improves overall health and can prevent or cure many diseases (Blair, 1995; Pate et al., 1995).
- Lower risk of heart attack and stroke, diabetes-type 2, metabolic syndrome, osteoporosis, and high cholesterol—exercise also increases HDL, or "good," cholesterol, like that found in plants, nuts, or fish like salmon or tuna, which helps rid the body of bad cholesterol and keeps blood flowing smoothly, making our hearts

stronger (Blair, 1995; Pate et al., 1995). Exercise not only prevents, but helps treat these diseases, as well (Griffin & Trinder, 1978; Helmrich et al., 1991).

- Lower overall cancer rates, especially colon and breast cancer—exercising at least four hours per week has been shown to lower the risk of breast cancer by 37% (Thune et al., 1997).
- Improved immune system for overall better health—better immune functioning means less illness, which benefits us physically and mentally (Northrup, 2006).
- Improved quality of sleep and greater energy—exercise delivers oxygen to the brain, body, and heart. This increases stamina to help us feel less fatigued during the day and sleep better at night, creating even greater energy (Driver & Taylor, 2000; Griffin & Trinder, 1978; Rodriguez, 2011).
- Increased muscle strength and mass, enhanced flexibility and movement, and stronger bones—exercise keeps our bones sturdy and our joints and muscles strong and limber. This helps us move and can lessen our risk for injury, especially as we age (Hunter et al., 2004; Williams et al., 2007; Nelson et al., 2007).
- Alleviated symptoms of premenstrual syndrome (PMS)—exercise can reduce cramping, bloating, and even mental and emotional symptoms of PMS in women (Prior, 1987).
- Regular exercise can increase your life expectancy by an average of seven years (Belloc and Breslow, 1972). One study in the *New England Journal of Medicine* showed that women who weren't fit had twice the risk of death than those who were (Gulati et al., 2005).

Bottom line: exercise is critical to a long, healthy life.

The Mental Health Benefits of Exercise

Exercise is also critical to a long, happy life. We can experience significant gains in all aspects of our mental health through exercise, including our emotional, intellectual, social, and even spiritual well-being.

Many may start exercising as a physical fitness goal—to lose weight, improve physical health, or "look good"—but as I often say, "We *keep* exercising for the mental health benefits." I know that's how it's been for me, and for so many of my clients. Once you understand and experience the mental health benefits of exercise for yourself, I am convinced you'll feel the same.

So what are the mental health benefits of exercise? Let's take a look. According to the research, exercise:

- increases levels of serotonin, dopamine, and norepinephrine in the brain. These neurotransmitters are typically low in people suffering from depression, anxiety, or other mental illnesses. Exercise works like a medication to improve and normalize neurotransmitter levels (Biddle & Fox, 1989; Chouloff, 1994, 1997).
- increases endorphins. Aerobic exercise releases these "feel good" chemicals into the body, which are associated with improved mood and energy (Durden-Smith, 1978; Riggs, 1981).
- enhances mood. Going for a walk when feeling fatigued and irritable, or lifting weights when feeling anxious, can reduce tension and increase energy to help us feel happier (Thayer, 2001). Exercise is definitely one of the quickest ways to improve mood.
- reduces and helps us manage stress, and leads to deeper relaxation. Exercise helps us calm down, rest, and relax more effectively, increasing our ability to withstand daily hassles and enabling us to manage stress more effectively (Mayo Clinic, 2012).
- lowers rates and symptoms of depression. Regular exercise has antidepressant effects that are as effective as psychotropic medications or psychotherapy for mild to moderate depression, making it a worthwhile adjunct, or even alternative, to traditional depression treatments. Exercise can even prevent major depression (Blumenthal et al., 2007, Smith et al., 2010; Leith, 2009).
- reduces anxiety and worries. Studies show exercise reduces, treats, and may even prevent anxiety and panic attacks. Strength

training has been shown to decrease tension and worry in the body and mind, and cardiovascular activity helps diminish worried or anxious thinking (Otto & Smits, 2011; Smits et al., 2008; Thayer 2001).

- improves mental clarity, efficiency, and cognitive functioning. We think more clearly when we exercise. This leads to increased learning, judgment, insight, and memory. Some studies have even shown that exercise is correlated with higher IQ scores (Young 1979; Gutin, 1966). Research shows that these gains continue in middle age and beyond (Singh-Manoux et al., 2005).

- enhances intuition, creativity, assertiveness, and enthusiasm for life. Exercise increases alpha waves, which are associated with stronger intuition and can lead to greater creativity (Northrup 2006). One study showed that walking during brainstorming rather than sitting at a desk boosts creativity by 60% (Oppezzo & Schwartz, 2014). Exercise also builds confidence and happiness, which in turn improves assertiveness and life satisfaction (Lannem et al., 2009; Valliant & Asu, 1985).

- improves quality of sexual intimacy. A healthy sex life is associated with better physical and mental health (Mayo Clinic, 2014), and exercise is associated with a healthier sex life.

- improved social health and relationships. Group or partner exercise increases social activity and connection while decreasing feelings of loneliness and isolation (Kulas, 2015). Exercising together as a couple or a family can improve and strengthen family relationships (we'll discuss this more in Key 3) (Ransdell et al., 2003).

- improves self-esteem and body image. Exercise makes us feel good about ourselves; not just about how we look, but even more so, about who we really are (we'll discuss this more in Key 2) (Sonstroem, 1984; Leith, 2009).

- increases spiritual connection. Walking, running, yoga, tai chi, and many other types of exercise are linked with increased spiritual awareness, energy, and connection (Musick et al., 2000). In fact, many people incorporate exercise into their spiritual practice (including me).

Overall, exercise is one of the best ways to improve mood and increase happiness and life satisfaction. It doesn't just make you healthier; exercise is key to living the life you desire. And, as we will see next, the benefits of exercise can reach even deeper: exercise can literally prevent, treat, and cure mental illness.

Exercise is Medicine

Were exercise available in a pill, *everyone* would take it. It's that good. Exercise functions like a medicine in the treatment of mental health disorders, and while there are various theories on how this works, the research is certain of one thing: it works.

Let's examine some of the more common mental health issues and what exercise can do to treat them. You may currently be struggling with one or more of these. Or, you may not. Chances are, however, that you, or someone you love, *will* experience at least one of these mental health conditions at some point in your life. So, pay close attention as we unfold the facts about the incredible impact of exercise on mental health disorders. It will not only continue to build the case for exercise, it will give you an idea of how exercise just might help you.

Stress and Burnout

Forty-four percent of Americans say they are more stressed now than they were five years ago. One in five experience extreme stress, including heart palpitations, panic, and depression. It is estimated that three out of four doctor's visits are stress-related, and 60% of all illness and disease is caused by stress (American Institute of Stress, 2015). Though stress is not a diagnosable disorder on its own, it definitely underlies and contributes to mental and physical health issues.

Many of us think of stress as a normal, daily occurrence. Family stress, occupational stress, financial stress—we see these as part of today's modern life, and therefore fail to seek stress-reduction or treatment. This is a mistake we can't afford to make because prolonged stress can lead to highly negative consequences for the body and mind, including headaches, muscular and joint pain, irritable bowel syndrome, ulcers, heart disease, depression, anxiety, insomnia, and a multitude of other mental and physical disorders (University of Maryland Medical Center, 2013). The personal cost of stress is high, though many fail to realize it. Stress defeats our health as well as our ability to manage mental and emotional issues.

Too much, or chronic, stress can eventually lead to burnout. Burnout occurs when our energy is gradually depleted, leading to reduced commitment and motivation—at work, at home, in relationships, or just in general. When we're burned out, we're less able to deal with life. Even small things can feel overwhelming, and every day can feel like a chore. Unchecked, burnout can progress to physical or mental illness like major depression or an anxiety disorder. One study, by the Mayo Clinic, showed that high stress at work, or occupational burnout, was associated with greater incidences of fatigue, illness, substance abuse, insomnia, and depression (Belluck, 2009).

Stress and Exercise

Exercise is one of the healthiest and most effective ways to treat short-term and chronic stress. It gets our mind off life's stressors, improves mood with natural feel-good chemicals, relieves tension, and increases mental clarity. Exercise also has the potential to reduce occupational and financial stress and prevent burnout (Gerber at al., 2013), and it's been shown to prevent the development of physical and mental illnesses, like depression, that often follow chronic stress.

One of the best things we can do when we're feeling stressed is to get moving. Go for a brisk walk, do some light housecleaning, or work in your garden. Whatever you can do to put your body in motion, do that. Exercise can clear your head, boost your energy, and help you deal with stress more effectively, in many cases helping you choose to simply let it go. (More on how to increase motivation, change your thinking, and overcome roadblocks to exercise in keys 4 through 6.)

Depression

Depression is one of the most common mental illnesses in the United States, with an estimated 16 million adults experiencing at least one major depressive episode in 2012 alone (NIMH, 2015b). Approximately 6.7% of American adults are clinically depressed in any given year (Kessler et al., 2009), 17% will experience a major depressive episode in their lifetime, and about half of those will experience recurring episodes of depression (Eaton et al., 2008).

Women tend to experience depression almost twice as often (11. 7%) as men (5.6%) (Centers for Disease Control and Prevention [CDC], n.d.), and depression affects approximately 15% of postpartum women and 10% of pregnant women (PSI, 2015), as well as an estimated 10% of postpartum men worldwide and 14% of American men (Paulson et al., 2010). It is estimated that 1 in 33 children and 1 in 8 adolescents are also clinically depressed (Depression and Bipolar Support Alliance [DBSA], 2015).

Symptoms of clinical depression include: sadness, fatigue, poor concentration, changes in appetite and/or sleep, loss of interest in activities one used to enjoy, feelings of hopelessness or helplessness, possible suicidal thoughts/intentions, and a negative view of oneself, the future, and the world. Depression often coincides with, or leads to, a host of other physical and mental disorders, including cancer, heart attacks, stroke, diabetes, eating disorders, and substance abuse (DBSA, 2015). Globally, depression is considered the third most important cause of disease burden and ranks first in higher and middle-income countries (WHO, 2008). Most startlingly, though, the WHO has predicted that depression will be the leading cause of death, second only to heart disease, by the year 2020 (Murray & Lopez, 1997).

Depression Treatment

Considering how prevalent and debilitating major depression can be, it's essential that those who suffer have valid and healthy treatment options. Depression is highly treatable, with an 80% success rate within four to six weeks for those who seek treatment through antidepressants, psychotherapy, support groups, or a combination of these (DBSA, 2015). Light therapy—sitting in bright morning light or in front of a light box for 30 or more minutes each day—has also been shown as a valid treatment for depression, seasonal affective disorder (SAD), and postpartum depression (Terman & Terman, 2005). For severe or treatment-resistant depression, electro-convulsive therapy, or ECT, is another effective option (Pagnin et al, 2004) and is considered one of the fastest ways to relieve depression, which is especially beneficial in severely depressed or suicidal individuals (Goldberg, 2014). While each of these treatments have been proven effective, only one in three of those suffering from depression will actually seek treatment or receive proper care (DBSA, 2015).

Depression and Exercise

Research shows that exercise is equivalent or superior to antidepressants in the treatment of both clinical (Blumenthal et al., 2007) and nonclinical depression. Exercise has also been shown to work as well as psychotherapy in treating mild to moderate depression. Regular exercise has been shown to cut depression prevalence in half—from 1 in 6 adults to 1 in 12 (Goodwin, 2003).

This is great news for those who don't seem to respond to traditional depression treatments, as well as for those who do respond. Exercise complements, and in many cases improves, the efficacy of these treatments (Leith, 2009), making exercise an outstanding alternative or addition to traditional treatment methods. Outdoor exercise adds the extra benefit of natural light therapy, bringing even greater benefits to those suffering from depression.

Anxiety

Many consider depression the most common mental illness in the United States, but while depression is certainly prevalent, anxiety is even more so. Anxiety disorders include phobias, social anxiety, panic disorder, generalized anxiety disorder, OCD, PTSD, and separation anxiety disorder, and are considered the most commonly occurring class of mental disorders (CDC, 2015).

Approximately 40 million adults suffer from clinical anxiety in the United States alone. Globally, developed countries exhibit higher yearly rates of clinical anxiety (10.4%) than developing countries (5.3%). Most anxiety disorders occur more frequently in women than in men (Baxter et al., 2013). Anxiety is actually the most common mental health disorder in women, affecting one in three throughout their lifespan. Anxiety disorders also affect many pregnant and postpartum women, with 3% to 5% experiencing postpartum OCD, 6% experiencing postpartum PTSD, and up to 10% experiencing postpartum panic disorder (PSI, 2015).

Anxiety Treatment

Anxiety typically develops as a result of several combined risk factors, including brain chemistry, genetics, personality, life events, and even hormones or other biochemical shifts. Because of this, it's important to focus on both biological and psychological factors when treating anxiety. Anxiety disorders, similar to depression, are highly treatable, and traditional treatment involves antianxiety medications and psychotherapy, especially CBT.

However, also like depression, anxiety often goes untreated. Only about one-third of those suffering from anxiety actually seek treatment (Anxiety and Depression Association of America [ADAA], 2014). One reason for this is that many believe anxiety is a "normal" part of life. It isn't until anxiety reaches high clinical levels, or becomes debilitating, that many seek help. Those suffering from anxiety are three to five times more likely to go to the doctor for health concerns and six times more likely to be hospitalized for mental illness than those without an anxiety disorder (ADAA, 2014).

Another reason for untreated anxiety is stigma. Many may feel it's easier to say we have a physical health problem (i.e. heart trouble) than to admit the problem may stem from psychological causes (i.e. panic attacks). This leads to misdiagnosis and thus mistreatment of anxiety disorders. It's just one of the many unfortunate consequences of the stigma that continues to stalk mental illness.

Anxiety and Exercise

Exercise is a helpful solution for anxiety disorders because it can treat the symptoms of anxiety with or without a firm diagnosis or the addition of other, traditional treatments. Exercise has been shown to decrease overall anxiety levels by reducing muscle tension, lowering blood pressure and heart rate, and producing a tranquilizing effect through increasing alpha waves in the brain (Leith, 2009). Once again, exercise is literally like medicine in the treatment of anxiety.

Unfortunately, many experiencing anxiety struggle to stick with an exercise program because the physical sensations involved in increased activity can mimic the physical sensations involved in anxiety disorders. This may lead anxiety sufferers to feel highly uncomfortable or even fear their body's response to exercise. High intensity or competitive exercise can actually increase symptoms of anxiety in some. It is therefore recommended that those seeking anxiety relief focus on moderate intensity, non-competitive exercises, like walking, running, swimming, weight-training, and other rhythmic exercises that incorporate large muscle groups (Leith, 2009). We will discuss this more in Key 6, but for now it's important to know that over time, and with great patience and love, anxiety-sufferers can adapt and adjust to exercise. They can begin to experience the calming pay-off of exercise and even learn to enjoy it.

In addition to treating general anxiety, studies also show exercise can significantly improve symptoms of various specific anxiety disorders, including panic disorder, OCD, PTSD, and social anxiety disorder.

- A comprehensive review of the research on anxiety disorders and exercise found that most studies focused on panic disorder. They found that, though some patients with panic disorder phobically avoid exercise, many do not, and that acute and long-term exercise are not only safe for those suffering from panic disorder, they significantly reduce anxiety symptoms (O'Connor, Raglin, & Martinsen, 2000). Another study comparing exercise to placebo and antianxiety drug treatments found that, though dropout rates were significantly higher for the exercise (31%) and placebo (27%) groups compared to the drug treatment group (0%), both exercise and antianxiety medication significantly decreased symptoms of panic disorder. The drug intervention worked more quickly and effectively; however, both lowered anxiety levels and also decreased associated symptoms of depression (Brooks et al., 1998).
- In a study of those diagnosed with OCD, participants reported less negative mood and anxiety symptoms following exercise; and, over time, those who stuck with their exercise routine reported less frequent episodes of obsessions and compulsions (Abrantes et al., 2009).
- Research has shown that those suffering from PTSD tend to be more sedentary and experience greater physical health concerns. Exercise has been proven to decrease sedentary behavior, improve body composition, improve quality of sleep, and treat the spectrum of symptoms, including depression, that accompany PTSD (Rosenbaum et al., 2011).
- For those struggling with social anxiety disorder, aerobic exercise has been shown to reduce clinical anxiety symptoms while simultaneously increasing a sense of well-being. These benefits appear not only during the intervention phase, but last up to three months later (Jazeiri et al., 2012).

Bipolar Disorder

Bipolar disorder is less common than anxiety and depression, with a reported lifetime prevalence rate of 4%. However, for those suffering, managing bipolar disorder can be particularly challenging.

Bipolar disorder consists of episodes of mania or hypomania in which the person feels speeded up, sleeps less, and tends to engage in harmful or unhelpful behaviors, followed by episodes of deep depression. In bipolar I disorder, the mania is generally more intense, lasts longer, and has more serious and obvious symptoms, while bipolar II disorder includes hypomanic episodes that are less intense. Because the symptoms of hypomania in bipolar II disorder tend to be less noticeable or harmful than those in bipolar I, it has often been called the "depression imposter." Many are consequently misdiagnosed with unipolar depression because they don't seek help during the hypomanic phases, not seeing them as a problem. It often isn't until the depressive episode hits that the sufferer finally seeks help. When the person finally does seek help, the medical or mental health provider may recognize the depression yet fail to investigate the possibility of a previous manic or hypomanic episode, resulting in a misdiagnosis of major depressive disorder. It only takes one manic or hypomanic episode to place an individual on the bipolar spectrum, and thus it's easy to see how this diagnosis may be missed. This can especially be a problem if the patient is placed on antidepressant medications, which can aggravate mania and worsen the bipolar illness.

Bipolar disorders, types I and II, are considered the most expensive mental health disorder, costing nearly twice as much as depression, per person. They are also associated with greater consequences, such as reduced work productivity, increased time away, more incidences of hospitalization, and greater impact on quality of life (CDC, 2015). Bipolar disorder, like anxiety and depression, is more common in women than in men, with a three-to-two ratio. It tends to have an earlier age of onset for men than women, however, with a median onset age of 25 years old.

Women who suffer from bipolar disorder are at a high risk of developing a pregnancy/postpartum mood or anxiety disorder, especially postpartum psychosis. Postpartum psychosis affects one in every one thousand new mothers and is a serious, potentially life-threatening illness for mother and baby. Those diagnosed with postpartum psychosis, in turn, almost always end up with a diagnosis of bipolar disorder. It is therefore imperative for women suffering from bipolar disorder to seek appropriate mental and physical health care when considering pregnancy. (We'll address pregnancy and postpartum mental health more in Key 3.)

Bipolar Disorder Treatment

Bipolar disorder requires lifelong treatment and maintenance, but with appropriate care, those with bipolar disorders may live a relatively normal lifestyle. Medication is considered the first line of treatment for bipolar disorder, including mood stabilizers, antipsychotics, antidepressants, and/or antianxiety medications. Psychotherapy, individually or in couples or family therapy, is also helpful in teaching those with bipolar disorder to manage their symptoms, learn healthy coping strategies, and work through relationships and other issues related to their illness. Cognitive-behavioral therapy is one of the most highly recommended forms of therapy for bipolar disorder. (More on CBT in Key 5).) ECT has also been shown to effectively reduce symptoms of mania and may additionally be utilized to reduce the often-severe depressive symptoms that accompany bipolar disorder (Pagnin 2004, Goldberg 2014).

Bipolar Disorder and Exercise

Considering the pervasive, intense nature of bipolar disorder and its treatment, one would think exercise would be more commonly recommended. Research shows that structured exercise can improve emotional, thought-related, and physical symptoms in patients with bipolar disorder. It can help calm the mind during manic or hypomanic phases, improving thought clarity, judgment, and insight. Also, the mood-enhancing and anti-inflammatory effects of exercise seem particularly helpful in alleviating depressive symptoms in those suffering from bipolar disorder (Mohammed et. al., 2009).

Additionally, considering the common misdiagnosis of bipolar II disorder as depression, and the consequential trouble often caused by misprescribed antidepressants, exercise seems a safe, healthy alternative or addition to treatment. There are no known negative side effects of exercise on bipolar disorder, and considering the many positive gains, it seems a logical solution to add exercise as an important treatment recommendation.

Schizophrenia

Schizophrenia affects about 1% of the population. It is a serious thought disorder and is associated with a high risk for suicide. About one-third of those suffering from schizophrenia will attempt suicide and 1 in 10 will eventually take their own lives (CDC, 2015). Schizophrenia is also associated with co-occurring physical and mental health issues, higher unemployment rates, and poorer life skills.

Schizophrenia, unlike anxiety and depression, affects more men than women. Men also tend to have a younger average age of onset, 21, than women, 27. Nine out of 10 men with schizophrenia will manifest symptoms before age 30, compare to 2 in 10 women (CDC, 2015).

Schizophrenia Treatment

Treatment for schizophrenia includes antipsychotic and/or mood-stabilizing medications and often includes frequent hospitalization to stabilize the patient. Psychotherapy and social support have also been shown to help those with schizophrenia, but treatment adherence rates are low with this disorder because of the severe thought and behavior-related symptoms.

Schizophrenia and Exercise

Considering the magnitude of schizophrenia and the challenges of medication and therapy adherence, exercise is a worthy option to examine. Research shows exercise improves mental clarity and helps those suffering from schizophrenia feel less overwhelmed by their symptoms. Exercise can alleviate depression and anxiety symptoms in those with schizophrenia, and also works to calm symptoms like auditory hallucinations (Faulkner & Biddle, 1999; Gorczynski & Faulkner, 2010). Exercise has also been shown to improve physical health and well-being in schizophrenic individuals (Bernhard & Ninot, 2012).

One thing to consider is that exercise, like medication and therapy, also requires adherence, and this may be a downside with schizophrenic individuals. However, research shows it is definitely possible for those living with schizophrenia to stick with an exercise program. Learning strategies to maintain regular exercise and overcome blocks that prevent exercise, as we will discuss in the keys to come, would undeniably benefit schizophrenic individuals.

Drug and Alcohol Addiction

It's estimated that 22.1 million people in the United States over age 12 (8.9% of the population), meet the criteria for a drug or alcohol addiction (Substance Abuse and Mental Health Services Administration [SAMHSA], 2015). Addiction occurs when a person develops a pattern of behavior in which they: 1) use a substance over and over, 2) become tolerant to the effects of that substance, and 3) experience withdrawal symptoms when trying to quit. According to the American Society of Addiction Medicine (ASAM) (2011), those in the grips of addiction experience the following:

1. Inability to **A**bstain from the substance/process
2. Impaired **B**ehavioral control
3. Constant **C**raving for the drug/alcohol/behavior—they can't stop thinking about it; their body hungers for it

4. Diminished recognition of how the substance/process is impacting their behavior, loved ones, relationships, work, and life

5. Dysfunctional Emotional responses to situations, people, and oneself

Addictions are believed to activate the brain's reward system, leading to feelings of euphoria or pleasure that become so pronounced that addicts ignore normal responsibilities and life activities. Addiction has also been shown to cause significant impairment in executive functioning—one's ability to plan, perceive, learn, control impulses, and have healthy insight and judgment (ASAM, 2011). Consequently, addiction causes significant distress or life impairment, including health, work, relationship, and legal issues. There is also a high rate of crossover among addicted individuals, with many being addicted to multiple substances and/or processes at once (Sussman et al., 2011).

It's estimated that 2-3% of the population has a process, or behavioral addiction—like gambling, internet addiction, social media, online gaming, food, sex, viewing pornography, and even exercise (Sussman et al., 2011). (We'll address exercise addiction below.) Many believe these numbers to be even higher, though research and statistics are currently hard to come by for process addictions as a whole. Internet addiction rates in the United States and Europe are estimated to fall between 1.5% and 8.2% of the population (Cash et al., 2012), and it's believed that as many as 1 in 25 adults is affected by compulsive sexual behavior or obsessions with sex-related thoughts, feelings, or behaviors that they cannot seem to control (University of Cambridge, 2014). One important study at the University of Cambridge (2014) took a deeper look and found that those suffering from sex addiction, or compulsive sexual behavior, experienced similar brain activity when viewing pornographic images as drug addicts experience when abusing drugs. Considering that 25% of all search engine requests are pornography-related, totaling 68 million searches per day (Smith, 2015), the potential for developing these kinds of process addictions is great. Compulsive behaviors, such as overeating, gambling, and watching porn to excess, are becoming more and more common and are associated with neurological complications, social troubles, and psychological distress (Cash et al., 2012). In fact, one of the primary characteristics of addiction—to substances or processes—is that the person continues to use or engage in the behavior despite serious negative consequences.

This speaks to the power of addictions of all types. Drug, alcohol, and behavioral addictions—they are a rampant problem in our society. We need awareness, education, and healthy prevention and treatment options to curb the growing problem of addiction.

Addiction Treatment, and Exercise

Addiction can become life threatening, thus treatment must be taken seriously, typically focusing on a lifelong recovery process. The best addiction treatment programs involve several components, including self-management, social support/support groups, and professional care by those trained in the treatment of the specific substance or behavior.

Exercise is a valuable addition to addiction treatment programs for many reasons (Faulkner & Biddle, 1999). First, it has been shown to improve sleep and mental clarity, which lead to better decision-making. Second, as we know, exercise can reduce depression and anxiety, which are common underlying factors that lead people to self-medicate with substances/processes. Third, the mood-enhancing effects of exercise may also mimic the effects of addictive substances in a healthy way, leading to a decreased need for the substance/process and a lower risk of relapse (Alcoholrehab. com, 2015; Taylor et al., 1985).

Because exercise helps the brain and body in such powerful ways, it may also serve as a preventative measure for those at risk for drug, alcohol, or process addictions. The National Institute on Drug Abuse actually put forth $4.3 million to study this possibility and found that the benefits exercise has on the brain may be important in strengthening young people against addictions. One study found that high school students who exercise regularly are less likely to smoke marijuana or nicotine, and those who are involved in sports also have less likelihood of developing addictions, perhaps because of the physical and mental health benefits of exercise as well as the involvement of positive role models in their lives, like coaches and teachers (Volkow, 2011).

Whatever the causes, it's clear: helping young people get out and move, engage in sports, or regularly participate in other physical activities is not only a healthy substitute for processes, behaviors, and substances that may be addictive, but it is also valuable in the mental and physical prevention of addictions.

A Note about Exercise Addiction

Because it is common for addicts to replace one addiction with another, exercise addiction is something to watch out for. Exercise addiction is real and can present a serious risk to physical and mental health. The cause of exercise addiction varies, but in general it's believed that, similar to drug, alcohol, or other process addictions, the person becomes dependent upon the positive feelings exercise offers. Exercise addiction may also include a strong need for "control" over one's body or life in general, and often points to an underlying anxiety disorder, such as an eating disorder or OCD (Recovery.org, 2015). However, as we will see, the underlying anxiety and the exercise addiction itself may improve with healthy, regular exercise, not because of the physical changes so much as the mental health benefits exercise provides. (We'll discuss overcoming exercise addiction more in Key 6.)

Eating Disorders, Body Image, and Exercise

Exercise has been mostly ignored as a "medicine" for eating disorders in the past, due to its relationship with the disease itself. It is true, those who struggle with eating disorders often use exercise as a way to control weight. However, recent research shows exercise can be beneficial. Exercise can lead to improvements in physical appearance and body image, but it's not the physical benefits of exercise that make the difference with eating disordered individuals—it's the mental health benefits (Cook et al., 2011).

Eating disorders tend to involve a high level of underlying anxiety and are also often linked with OCD. We've already discussed the many ways exercise can treat anxiety. The same works for eating disorders. Exercise improves relaxation, lowers tension and worry, and improves mood, all of which can improve eating disorders. The effects exercise can have on self-esteem and depression can also reduce the risk of, or help treat, eating disorders (Cook et al., 2011).

Personality Disorders and Exercise

Personality disorders—including narcissistic, borderline, dependent, and histrionic, to name a few—are pervasive and invasive. They're hard to treat because they're so ingrained into a person's way of being in the world, and often, those suffering don't feel they need help.

Though the evidence produces mixed results about exercise's ability to improve personality disorders, there are studies that show positive benefits from exercise. For those who learn to manage and stick with an exercise routine, exercise is associated with improved insight, judgment, and mental clarity, all of which alleviate the more intense symptoms of personality disorders. Exercise can also treat underlying conditions, like anxiety or depression, which can worsen personality disorders. Finally, exercise has the potential to positively impact and even improve personality traits, like sociability, internal motivation, assertiveness, neuroticism, placidity, emotional stability, and self-confidence (University of Minnesota Deluth, n.d.). This is great news for those of us who might like to improve a thing or two about our personality: exercise may be the key.

Cognitive Decline, Dementia, and Exercise

Alzheimer's disease is the sixth leading cause of death in the United States and the fifth leading cause for those older than 65. Approximately 5.3 million Americans are currently diagnosed with

Alzheimer's, and that number is expected to more than double by 2050 (CDC, 2015).

Exercise earlier in life has been shown to prevent cognitive decline later in life, improving mental clarity and functioning and keeping the body and mind healthier and more vibrant (Larson et al., 2006). Aerobic exercise has also been shown to increase oxygen flow to the brain and thereby decrease brain cell loss in the elderly. Additional benefits may be gained from engaging in physical activities that also involve focus, planning, or thinking. Exercising with another person is also great for social health, especially in the elderly (Alzheimer's Association, 2015b).

The good news is it's not necessary to exercise vigorously to obtain these benefits against cognitive decline; it's just necessary to get moving, and do so regularly.

Grief and Exercise

Loss and grief is a universal experience. If you haven't felt the sting of grief yet, hold tight, because eventually you will. Loss comes in many forms, including death, but also divorce, job loss, financial loss, infertility, loss of dreams or what you thought would be, and many others. Grief is a normal part of losing someone or some-thing you care for, and though this type of grief is not considered a mental health disorder, it can be a difficult experience to go through. Many people try to ignore, deny, or stuff grief, failing to acknowledge their emotional needs. Some become so over-whelmed by grief that they stay stuck in it for years, feeling unable to move forward. This can not only significantly impact the griev-er's relationships and life, but also can develop into pathological grief, which requires psychological treatment.

It's estimated that approximately 10-20% of the bereaved meet the criteria for what is known as complicated grief. Complicated grief is pathological grief that often occurs when those with a his-tory of depression, anxiety, or other mental illness lose someone who was very important in their life. Symptoms include an intense longing for the deceased, preoccupation with thoughts or images of them, deep, relentless sadness, guilt, or anger, avoidance of people, places or situations that trigger memories of the deceased, and difficulty moving forward with positive relationships and emotions (Shear, 2010).

Whether grief is normal or complicated, we must grieve our losses, and one way to process grief involves physical activity. Research shows exercise helps get us out of our own head. Endorphins help with the depression and sadness of grief, and getting outside in the sunlight and seeing people remind us of the good in the world around us. Exercise also increases self-confidence, to help us feel more in control of life again. Yes, exercise is one important thing we can do to overcome grief (Wellness Monthly, 2012). (We'll explore more on overcoming grief in Key 2.)

Other Mental Health Stressors that May Benefit from Exercise

Though we've touched on some of the more prominent mental health concerns, there are many others that have been shown to benefit from exercise as well.

Bad Moods

We've all had our share of bad days—days when our mood just isn't what we'd like it to be. Exercise is one of the best things we can do for a bad mood. Not only does it give us much-needed energy and mental clarity, studies show that regular exercise is an even more powerful and effective treatment for reducing negative mood than even relaxation techniques or other enjoyable, distracting activities (North et al., 1990). Further, research shows that cardiovascular activity is ideal for improving negative moods related to low energy, whereas weight-lifting or strength-training is most effective for negative moods related to stress, tension, or anxiety (Thayer, 2001).

Chronic Illness

Those suffering from chronic illnesses like cardiovascular disease, fibromyalgia, and Parkinson's disease have been shown to benefit from exercise. First, it can improve the physical symptoms of many illnesses and lower cholesterol and blood pressure, strengthening the heart and sending more blood and oxygen to the brain and body, building needed muscle and controlling weight. Exercise also decreases the depressive symptoms often associated with chronic illness. Over time, exercise may help reduce the need for medications. It also decreases stress, improves relaxation, and combats the inactivity that so commonly accompanies many illnesses (Herring et al., 2012). Furthermore, even leisure time physical activity is clearly associated with mortality risk reduction, including cardiovascular- and cancer-related deaths (Araujo & Stein, 2015).

Chronic Pain

Supervised, individually designed programs that incorporate stretching and muscle strengthening exercises can improve chronic pain (Hayden et al., 2005). Though adherence can be a problem when pain is involved, studies show that, overall, exercise is safe for individuals with ailments such as chronic back pain and that it can increase back flexibility and strength. Studies also show that exercise can reduce the cognitive, affective, behavioral, and disability components of conditions like chronic back pain (Rainville et al., 2004).

Couples and Family Relationship Struggles

Relationship issues are one of the most common mental health struggles in the world, affecting all of us at some point. Exercising together has been shown to strengthen family relationships of all types, and it can help you tackle relationship problems and increase intimacy, too. Couples who exercise together not only spend more time together, but they also tend to have healthier communication, especially when they use exercise time to talk about work, family, and their relationship. Studies show that working out with your partner may even enhance exercise gains; because you're facing the challenge as a team, with someone you care about and who cares about you, you're more likely to feel happier, more motivated and supported, and to enjoy exercising more. Exercising together helps couples feel more grounded in their relationship, planting the seed that perhaps they can face other, more important things, together, as a team. It creates better bodies, minds, and relationships. Studies also show that parent-child relationships can be strengthened by exercising together. One study of previously sedentary mothers and daughters found that, after a 12-week program of mother-daughter exercise, both the home-based and university-based group mother and daughters agreed their relationship with their daughter/mother had improved as a result (Ransdell et al., 2003).

The list goes on. Exercise seems to have the potential to positively impact just about every mental health issue one may experience. And if the case hasn't been made clearly enough, then perhaps looking at the following case example will help.

How Exercise Works to Improve Mental Health

There are several different theories on how exercise improves mental health, and no one hypothesis seems to explain it all. Understanding a few of the main ideas of how exercise works, however, can help us better understand how exercise may work on our mental health, too.

The Endorphin Hypothesis

Endorphins are the "feel good" chemicals released in the brain when we exercise. These chemicals actually mimic the chemical structure of morphine and have the ability to ease pain, regulate emotion, and produce a sense of euphoria often referred to as "the runner's high." It is believed that this sense of euphoria is responsible for improving mental health by reducing depression, anxiety, and other negative mood states. This is perhaps the most popular theory, though the research behind it isn't particularly compelling (Leith, 2009).

The Monoamine Hypothesis

This theory posits that exercise improves mental health through changes in monoamines in the brain, like serotonin, dopamine, and norepinephrine. When neurotransmitters such as these become too low in the brain, emotional symptoms and mental distress or illness ensues. Many studies have produced evidence to support the idea that exercise increases levels of neurotransmitters in the brain, and thus, this hypothesis is compelling (Leith, 2009).

The Anti-inflammatory Theory

Anti-inflammatories are associated with greater heart health, lower depression, and improved aging, and exercise is a natural anti-inflammatory. Simply engaging in active leisure time activities has been shown to have anti-inflammatory effects. Those who exercise regularly were reported in one study to have lower inflammation markers even 10 years later (Hamer et al., 2012).

Other theories include: self-efficacy theory (when we believe we can achieve something and do it, we feel better about ourselves, and this improves our mental health); the thermogenic hypothesis (when we increase our body temperature through exercise, it results in the deeper slow wave sleep that makes us feel relaxed and renewed); and the distraction hypothesis (when we're distracted from stress, or get a "time out" through exercise, we feel mentally refreshed and improved) (Leith, 2009).

Whatever the reasons, the evidence is solid: exercise works. It can significantly improve our mental health and, consequently, our life satisfaction. But it's up to us to take advantage of it.

Let's look at a real-life example of the power of exercise for mental health.

Surviving to Thriving: Mechelle's Story

Mechelle found her world crashing down when her marriage of over 20 years was suddenly over. Her finances were in shambles, her three children were struggling, and she was battling self-doubt, fear, and pain. Every time she recalled her soon-to-be ex's words, "You'll never be able to do this on your own," she clinched her jaw, and developed significant tooth pain as a result. Depression set in deeply. "It wrapped its lonely fingers tightly around me," she said, "squeezing my very soul."

Mechelle spent the next few months afraid to get out of bed. She didn't want to move. She wanted to lie there and hide from all the responsibilities that tore at her. As she lay in bed one morning, her puffy eyes were drawn to the corner of her room. In the sunlight, she saw the pink laces of her running shoes, "stretching across the carpet, reaching toward me. Calling me," she said. For a week, they called as she lay in bed, and for a week, she turned away from them. Rolling over was the only exercise she was getting. Until one day, when her son came home from wrestling practice full of energy and happiness. "I wanted what he was feeling," Mechelle said. "That's when my eyes finally focused on those pink laces."

In an attempt to calm the negative voices in her head, Mechelle told herself she would only run to the mailbox and back. And she did. Not one step farther. That little jog to the mailbox started something. It changed her day. She felt a small glimpse of what her son had shown her, and she wanted more. That night, she wrote down a goal of running to the end of the block, and the next day, she did. Writing down her running goals became a nightly ritual, and waking to those written goals sitting next to her alarm clock reminded her of the high she felt when running. It pushed her up and out once more—day after day, week after week.

It wasn't easy, and there were plenty of times when Mechelle found herself on her knees in the middle of the forest, sobbing and screaming in pain and grief. Other times, she couldn't take another step because of paralyzing emotional pain, so she would just fall and let the pain in. As she learned to feel the emotional pain, she began to learn to calm herself, to trust herself, and eventually, to believe in herself enough to face her fears.

"A funny thing happened after a few months," Mechelle says. "The tears stopped. I had looked pain in the face, shaken its hand, and found that it was something I could deal with. As I faced my pain, I overcame my fear. Then, I got busy empowering myself." Mechelle began to work on changing her thoughts, and turning the negative self-talk into positive mantras and affirmations. "This positive self-talk became as much a part of my run as lacing up my shoes," she said. "I would repeat the words over and over on the dusty trails. One foot, 'brave.' The next, 'strong.' And the next step pounded, 'competent.'"

Those are Mechelle's truths today. "I am brave, strong, and competent. It has been years since I left that toxic situation, and not only am I a happy, productive person moving forth with dignity and grace, but so are my kids. We are not surviving. We are thriving. And my teeth? They no longer hurt and can be seen easily, as I smile on my new life."

Exercise for Mental Health = Exercise for Life

Look what exercise has done for Mechelle, and for her family. What could exercise do for you?

Exercise may be the best thing we can do for our emotional, mental, physical, social, and spiritual well-being. It is surely one of the safest, simplest, most effective ways to treat and prevent mental illness, literally acting as medicine. This is the power of exercise for mental health: the power to heal your body and mind; and the power to protect and empower you, your whole life long.

Reflection Questions: Exercise and Mental Health

1. Review and consider all the exercise benefits, outlined above. Which appeal most to you? Highlight those you most desire to receive, and then write them below or copy them into your journal or notebook.

_____

_____

_____

_____

_____

_____

_____

_____

2. Reflect on a time when you felt good after being physically active. This may include any physical activity you did, for any amount of time, from any time of your life. Maybe it was after dancing when you were a child, weight lifting for a college physical education course, or playing a sport with friends last week. Whatever it was, hold it in your mind and try to remember how you felt at that time.

   a. Describe the activity with as many details as you can recall.

   _____

   _____

   _____

   _____

   _____

   b. What mental or physical health benefits did you experience after you were done? Did you feel energized, happier, or more self-confident? Did you sleep better, feel more relaxed, or have a less stressful day afterward? List as many as you can identify, and if it's only one thing, well, that's okay too.

_____

_____

_____

_____

_____

_____

c. What contributed to your sense of feeling good after exercising? Was it being with friends, being in nature, or doing something you enjoy? Identify as many things as you can that helped motivate you to exercise and contributed to your positive experience.

_____

_____

_____

_____

_____

_____

_____

_____

(If you can't think of anything at first, keep thinking. Even if it is a distant memory, chances are you've had at least one positive experience. If you still can't, then stick with me. The rest of this book will help you learn how to feel good after exercise. That's what it's all about.)

3. Create a list of all the benefits of exercise you have previously experienced using what you wrote in items one and two. Then, as we move through the remainder of the keys, continue to add to your list of exercise benefits. Refer to

this list whenever you need to be reminded of why you're doing this work; it will keep you motivated to exercise for mental health, and for life.

_____

_____

_____

_____

_____

_____

_____

_____

_____

_____

_____

_____

_____

_____

_____

_____

_____

_____

_____

_____

_____

_____

_____

_____

_____

_____

_____

IMPROVE YOUR SELF-ESTEEM
WITH EXERCISE

"To be beautiful means to be yourself. You don't need to be accepted by others. You need to accept yourself."

—Thich Nhat Hanh

Most experts see self-esteem as an important aspect of mental health. I agree: self-esteem seems to underlie almost every issue for which my clients come to therapy. They say they're there because of depression, or anxiety, or relationship problems, but at its core, the real problem is almost always a struggle with self-esteem.

Self-esteem can be defined as the opinion we have of ourselves, or how we feel about ourselves. Healthy self-esteem means we have a positive outlook about ourselves, others, and life. The world calls this "high self-esteem," and it is associated with healthier behavior, including greater independence, leadership, life adaptability, resilience to stress (Fox, 2000), more sports involvement and exercise, healthier diet, less smoking, and lower suicide risk (Torres & Fernandez, 1995).

On the other hand, "low self-esteem" is correlated with the absence of wellness and is a frequent underlying aspect of depression, anxiety, low assertiveness, feelings of hopelessness, suicidal ideation, and a poor sense of personal control (Fox, 2000). Low self-esteem is also associated with higher self-criticism, negative thinking, an inability to cope effectively with life, and poorer overall mental health, including a greater chance of developing clinical depression, anxiety, suicidal tendencies, eating disorders, stress, substance abuse, and other mental illnesses (Mann et al., 2004).

In fact, self-esteem is one of the strongest predictors of subjective well-being. It is an essential aspect of mental wellness and quality of life (Diener, 1984). Feeling good about who, and how, we are helps us feel good about life's situations and other people, and helps us face challenges with confidence and compassion. Healthy self-esteem is also correlated with greater physical activity, and greater physical activity is correlated with higher self-esteem (Fox, 2000). It's therefore crucial we develop healthy self-esteem if we want a rich, healthy, and happy life. As we'll discuss below, exercise can play a valuable role in helping us achieve this.

The Three Components of Mental Health

Self-esteem comes from our life experiences. For better or worse, our family, school, work, friends, and community shape our self-esteem from the time we're young. Self-esteem is also shaped by our experiences with our body and brain—brain chemistry, hormones, and other biological processes. These are what I call the three components of mental health: 1) brain chemistry, 2) hormones and biological influences, and 3) life experiences. When we struggle with any of these components, we tend to feel worse about ourselves, and we're more likely to suffer from low self-esteem.

Understanding the three components to mental health can be extremely valuable in helping people see that mental illness is not a "weakness," and that it usually involves much more than meets the eye. It has allowed me to help those struggling with depression, anxiety, bipolar disorder, and so forth, to understand *why*. "Why?" is a common question when it comes to mental health. "Why do I have depression?" "Why can't I just be 'strong enough' to shake this anxiety?" Understanding how these three components come together to create "earthquakes" in our mental health is one way to answer "why." Understanding "why" can be a big help when it comes to self-esteem. Before we move on, allow me to explain each component a little deeper.

The Brain

The brain we have today is not the same brain we had as children. Over time, it becomes altered by our physical and mental health, hormones and other chemical changes, and even life experiences. When we experience mental illness, it's a sign that the brain is struggling—that the neurotransmitters in the brain, like serotonin and dopamine, are not firing correctly. Psychotropic medications and psychotherapy help to correct these misfirings, and exercise works in the same way.

Hormones and Biological Influences

Hormones are the chemical messengers of the body. They are regulated by the pituitary, or master gland, which sends signals to other glands that then release hormones that regulate metabolism and mood, induce hunger and body temperature, prepare the body for the changes of puberty, childbirth, or menopause, control the reproductive cycle, and stimulate or inhibit growth. Because hormones affect such a wide variety of essential bodily processes, and because they are triggered in the brain and released into the bloodstream, it's no wonder that hormones can cause a wide range of emotional distress, especially when we're faced with huge hormonal shifts, like during puberty, pregnancy/ postpartum, and perimenopause. Hormones are also direct precursors to the neurotransmitters in the brain that are associated with mental health. When hormones shift, neurotransmitters also shift. This can lead to sudden and dramatic changes in emotional or mental well-being, especially for those who are sensitive to hormonal shifts.

Life Experiences

Most of us fail to recognize the impact our life experiences have on our brain. Stress, trauma, loss, mental illness, family problems and upbringing—each of these directly impacts the brain, altering the brain chemistry. This can lead to the onset of mental illness and make hormonal shifts even more noticeable and difficult to bear.

The Earthquake

Together, these things pile up, causing stress to our brain and eventually leading to tremors, or an "earthquake," like a major mental disorder. Just like the ground shifts over time and eventually shifts so much an earthquake ensues, so does our brain. (I first learned about the earthquake metaphor from Sichel & Driscoll's [2000] excellent book and have adapted it to apply here.)

For example, when Jennifer was younger, her parents split up. It was hard on her and her two brothers, but she was "tough," she says, and so she carried on. As a teenager, Jennifer began to struggle with premenstrual syndrome. Her mood symptoms were a challenge each month, creating even more tension in her already tense home, and her older brothers only made matters worse when they teased her about it, calling her "crazy." Jennifer determined she would never be called crazy by anyone else again. In college, when Jennifer's beloved grandmother passed away, she was devastated. At first, she told herself it was "just grief," but as the months went by and her symptoms worsened, leading her to fail several college courses for the first time ever, Jennifer had to admit, perhaps, it was something else. Her parents sent her to counseling, and when she came to me, it was clear Jennifer was suffering from major depression. Jennifer did not want to be depressed, telling herself it was "weak," as if she'd failed in her goal to "never be crazy again." Jennifer needed a new way to see things, one that could strengthen her sense of self-worth and not defeat it.

As I explained the earthquake metaphor, I helped Jennifer see that her parents' divorce, coupled with her body's sensitivity to hormones, coupled with her self-esteem struggles and lack of support as a teenager, had changed her brain chemistry and predisposed her for mental health issues down the road. When her grandmother died—boom—that set off the earthquake. The ground had been shifting in her brain for years, and one more traumatic experience was all it took for everything to come crumbling down. Understanding this helped Jennifer accept her depression and let go of the idea that experiencing depression made her "weak." Once she could see the many facets that contributed to her emotional challenges, she could begin to accept them, and self-acceptance, as we are about to see, is a key element of self-worth.

Do This . . .

Visit http://www.exercise4mentalhealth.com and download a copy of "The Earthquake Assessment Chart" I've adapted from Sichel & Driscoll (1999), or use the copy provided. Using this chart, plot your life experiences, shifts in hormones, and changes in brain chemistry. Then, go back and look for patterns in these three components of mental health. See how these may have created tremors or earthquakes, like mental and emotional struggles, in your life. Plot these on the "outward appearance" line. Seek understanding of your earthquakes and tremors, using the three components of mental health to help you understand "why." (For a video example, visit http://www.exercise4mentalhealth.com.)

Earthquake Assessment Chart

Outward Appearance/ Functioning	
Brain Chemistry	
Life Stress/ Experiences	
Hormonal Events	
Age	

www.Exercise4MentalHealth.com

The Pursuit of Self-Esteem, a Myth

Now that I've explained the human need for self-esteem, allow me to present a challenge to it. The trouble with self-esteem is that the way we are taught to pursue it doesn't always work. I can't tell you how many clients I've seen who report that they've been trying to improve their self-esteem for years, yet still don't feel confident, valuable, and/or worthy. Their efforts have been magnanimous, but the results just haven't been there. *Why is this?* I wondered, and began a long path of self-esteem research, theory development, and experimentation.

If I have learned anything about self-esteem over the years, it's that we've been looking at it all wrong. We are taught to pursue self-esteem, but perhaps the pursuit of self-esteem is a myth. Self-esteem is the opinion or feeling we have about who we really are, but it's not who we really are. It's easy to get caught up in "trying to think more positively about ourselves," or "trying to feel more self-love," while failing to realize these are both simply by-products of something else. How can we truly love ourselves, think positively about and believe in ourselves, if we're not sure who we really are?

Perhaps we don't increase self-esteem by trying to increase self-esteem. Perhaps that's why so many of us still feel like we're "not good enough," despite years of reading about, learning about, and working diligently to have "high self-esteem." Perhaps, instead, self-esteem—or the feeling that we are loveable, worthy, and capable—can only be increased by going deep and discovering who we really are. Perhaps we increase self-esteem by increasing our sense of self-worth.

What is Self-Worth?

Each of us has the ability to do great things, feel loved, and achieve our highest potential—in exercise, health and wellness, and in all areas of life. This is self-worth. I define self-worth as: "the ability to comprehend and accept my true value—to understand I am more than my body, mind, emotions, and behaviors, to see myself as my Creator sees me, to accept this Divine love, and to learn to love myself in like manner" (Hibbert, 2015). When we tap into our deeper, truer, unchanging self, we exude self-worth and experience self-esteem.

Self-worth is natural, inborn, and given to all, and, unlike self-esteem, isn't merely about self-appraisal. On the contrary, it's about setting the evaluations and criticisms aside and seeing and embracing what *is*. Yes, though the world may use self-esteem and self-worth interchangeably, in my mind, they have very different meanings. It is only through uncovering self-worth that we may begin to experience self-esteem. Without a true sense of who we are, no amount of positive thinking or feeling, or even exercise, will make a difference.

Self-Worth, Self-Esteem, and Exercise

What does all this have to do with exercise and mental health? Considering the impact self-esteem and self-worth have on our mental health, and considering the impact exercise has on mental health, by the transitive property, it's no wonder that exercise is also associated with healthier self-esteem, and vice versa. Research shows that:

- physical activity significantly impacts a child's sense of competency and self-worth. Those who feel more family support in physical activity, or who are surrounded by active family/friends, are more likely to engage in sports and other physical activities (Let's Move, 2015).
- regular exercise can increase self-esteem, self-confidence, self-efficacy (or the belief we can be effective in our life), self-acceptance, and self-concept (how we view ourselves). When we exercise, we feel much more positive, loving, and confident about who we are (Cohen & Shamus, 2009).
- exercise also improves self-esteem and sense of self-worth by improving underlying mental health issues. Exercise decreases depression, anxiety, tension, and stress, which consequently boosts self-esteem (Cohen & Shamus, 2009).
- exercise increases self-esteem across the lifespan. Exercise promotes a sense of self-worth in children, adolescents, and young adults (Ekelend et al., 2004), and is particularly helpful for young and adolescent girls 11 years old and younger, helping them

develop greater self-confidence that lasts throughout their life (Schmalz et al., 2007). In middle age, exercise is correlated with increased physical self-perceptions, including higher ratings of fitness, health, appearance, self-worth, and overall mental well-being (Fox, 2000). Studies show that exercise also produces positive changes in sense of self-worth in older adults, raising physical self-esteem and increasing much-needed social health and support (Fox, 2000).

- women may have the greatest potential for increases in self-esteem related to exercise. Women tend to struggle more with self-worth than men, with lower initial self-report scores on self-confidence, body image, physical activity, and self-esteem. This may be why they show the greatest increases in self-esteem through exercise; they have the most to gain (Lirgg, 1991).
- overall, exercise has the most potential to increase self-esteem in anyone who has much to gain—including those in poor physical health, middle-aged to older adults who tend to be in poorer physical condition, the overweight and obese, and those suffering from depression and other mental health disorders (Fox, 2000).

Interestingly, however, regular exercise or participation in sports is only moderately associated with more positive body image and self-perceptions from adolescence on (Sonstroem, Speliotis, & Fava, 1992). Though exercise is clearly correlated with being trim and fit, being trim and fit is only weakly associated with positive body image and self-perceptions. Those who struggle with body image, especially women and those experiencing eating disorders or over-exercising, do not think more highly of themselves as a result of exercise (Fox, 2000), while those who are overweight or in poorer health seem to experience greater body image and self-perception benefits.

This is important. It shows that, for some issues like eating disorders, exercise addiction, and very low self-esteem, exercise is not the recommended first line of treatment. Instead, in such cases, it may be more beneficial to seek psychotherapy first, to work directly on self-esteem and sense of self-worth, then to add exercise when the foundation of self-worth is strong.

Which Comes First—Exercise or Self-esteem?

Researchers have long been asking, "Which comes first—self-esteem or exercise?" We know there is a high correlation between those who are physically active and healthy self-esteem. Common consensus is that this relationship goes both ways. Those who already have high self-esteem are more likely to exercise and participate in sports, especially those who feel confident in their physical abilities and appearance. On the flip side, those with lower self-esteem and physical self-perceptions, including those who suffer from depression, anxiety, and other mental health disorders, are less likely to engage in regular physical activity. However, this group has the most to gain from exercise, and research shows that regular exercise increases positive self-feelings and evaluations, meaning they feel more confident, capable, and healthy through regular exercise and activity, leading to higher overall self-esteem (Fox, 2000).

While research can't exactly pinpoint, it appears there are several mechanisms that lead to improved self-esteem from exercise. First, as we already know, exercise improves mood and enhances positive self-regard. This, in turn, seems to have a positive effect on self-esteem. Second, exercise can improve body image, satisfaction, and acceptance for some, which increases overall self-esteem. Third, exercise leads us to feel more physically competent, which may then improve how we feel about ourselves overall. Fourth, exercise helps us feel more in control of our appearance, health, and bodily functioning, which can increase a sense of self-efficacy. And finally, exercise, and especially group exercise, can improve relationships and increase a sense of belonging, which is important in the development of self-esteem (Fox, 2000).

Overall, it's likely that each of these factors interplay to create improvements in mind, body, and self-esteem. Since exercise helps us improve our physical, mental, emotional, social, and spiritual health, it makes sense that this would lead to a greater quality of life and improved sense of self-worth. When we stick with an exercise or fitness routine, we demonstrate motivation and dedication, both of which are associated with greater self-esteem and self-perceptions (Fox, 2000). Bottom line: no matter how it works, exercise and self-esteem go hand in hand.

Exercise, Self-Esteem, and Self-Worth

Why, then, if exercise holds so many secret ingredients for our mental health and well-being, is it only weakly correlated with how we perceive ourselves, especially our bodies? I have a theory. I believe this happens because too many of us still don't feel our self-worth. Even when the outward evidence says, "You're important! You're valuable! You're an amazing human being!" we don't believe it. We believe our own "evidence" instead, evidence we've collected through our whole lives via true or untrue thoughts, beliefs, and perceptions of experiences. This "evidence" says, "I'm not good enough."

One of the main problems with self-esteem is that it's mostly based on external sources. Research shows that basing our worth on external sources—like appearance, academic or physical performance, or approval from others—leads to greater anger, stress, relationship and academic problems, and higher alcohol and drug use and eating disorders (Crocker, 2002).

In contrast, those who base their worth on *internal*, constant sources, such as being a virtuous person or sticking to moral standards, tend to have greater success in life, including higher grades and lower likelihood of eating disorders and drug/alcohol use. In fact, students in one study who based their self-worth on outward sources, like academic performance, were found to have *poorer* self-esteem, even when their grades were higher than others (Crocker, 2002). This shows the power of having a true, deep sense of self-worth versus basing our worth on self-perceptions and self-esteem.

Understanding self-worth is crucial in exercise for mental health success; it helps us believe we can do it, stick with it, and reach our fullest mental and physical health potential. When we feel confident, we're not only more likely to exercise; we're more likely to let go of the self-perceptions and beliefs that hold us back and make us feel like a "failure." We're more likely to overcome the roadblocks, stop unhealthy thoughts and beliefs, and stay motivated and dedicated to exercise. As psychologist Nathaniel Branden writes, "The level of our [sense of self-worth] has profound consequences for every aspect of our existence: how we operate in the workplace, how we deal with people, how high we are likely to rise, how much we are likely to achieve—and in the personal realm, with whom we are likely to fall in love, how we interact with our spouse, children, and friends, what level of personal happiness we attain" (1995, p. 4-5). Yes, we need self-worth.

A New View of Self-Esteem: The Pyramid of Self-Worth

The Pyramid of Self-Worth is a model I created for uncovering, discovering, and embracing self-worth. It moves us from the thoughts, feelings, and self-evaluations of self-esteem to a deeper understanding of who we are and what we're capable of.

Self-worth, unlike self-esteem, is not something we "go out and get." It's not based on anyone's opinion of us, and it's not based on how we think or feel about ourselves. We all possess self-worth; we just have to dig through the years of people, experiences, and thoughts that have told us otherwise. Trust me, this is true. I've worked with many people on this, and I have never found someone who has no underlying self-worth. All I've seen is a whole lot of people who don't know how to dig down and tap in to that self-worth. The Pyramid of Self-Worth can help. Here's how it works.

There are three layers to The Pyramid of Self-Worth, as shown in the figure below: 1) self-awareness, 2) self-acceptance, and 3) self-love. Together, these three layers build self-worth. Let's explore each a little more.

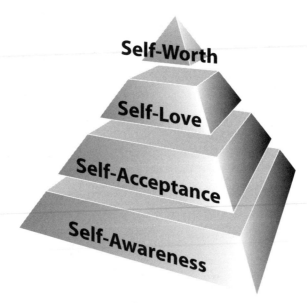

Fig. 1 The Pyramid of Self-Worth

Self-Awareness

Self-awareness means taking a bold, searching look at the good, the bad, the ugly, and the exceptional—what makes you unique, your talents, your highs and lows—to be willing to see it all, knowing everyone has strengths and weaknesses. It's hard to love or accept yourself if you don't know yourself. As we open up and examine who we really are—how we behave, what we think and believe, how we feel, what we're good at, and what we struggle with—then we can learn to accept it. And acceptance is critical to feeling self-worth.

It can be difficult to practice self-awareness at first, especially if you're not used to taking such an honest look at yourself. It can be hard to see your faults, and for many, even harder to see your strengths. When we're heading to the gym for the first time, for example, and see ourselves in the mirror, next to the mighty and fit, it can make us want to run and hide. But stick with it. Self-awareness is a miraculous tool, and the truth can truly set you free.

Do This . . . Self-Awareness

Using your journal, notebook, digital device, or this book, create two lists. The first is your list of strengths. What are you good at, especially when it comes to exercise and mental health? What do others tell you they like about you? What do you enjoy doing or feel you have to offer the world? Then, list your weaknesses. What do you struggle with, especially when it comes to exercise and mental health? What qualities would you like to overcome? We all have strengths and weaknesses, and learning to see them is the first step in learning to accept and embrace or overcome them.

My Strengths

_____

_____

_____

_____

_____

_____

My Weaknesses

_____

_____

_____

_____

_____

_____

Self-Acceptance

Once we see who and how we are, then we must learn to accept it. This is the toughest step for most and is usually a process that lasts a lifetime. When it comes to exercise and mental health we each possess certain strengths and weaknesses. Some are incredibly gifted athletically. Others have great willpower, motivation, or determination. Some struggle with physical strength, coordination, flexibility, or cardiovascular capacity. Others struggle with mental focus or self-confidence. Some exercise because they hate their body, but I'm hoping we can learn to love our bodies, and our minds, and appreciate the power we hold when we accept who we are and believe in who we have the potential to become.

Accept Weaknesses and Strengths

Self-acceptance is about seeing the truth and letting it be. Hard as it is, this is so important. As we learn to accept both our weaknesses and strengths, we begin to experience self-worth—independent of what we think, feel, do, or what others say about us. When we can say, "I know this is something I'm not good at, and I'm okay with that. I'm working on it," or "I am good at so many other things, I can let this one go," or even, "I'm not yet where I want to be, but I am going to fake it 'til I make it. I will not give up," well, that is self-worth speaking.

For some, it's more difficult to acknowledge and accept weaknesses. We think, irrationally, that having weaknesses makes us "weak." In fact, the opposite is true. Hiding and pretending to be someone we're not, getting stuck on other's opinions of us, and focusing too much on "self-esteem" is much weaker than getting real and embracing self-worth. *Acknowledging and accepting weakness is strength.* For example, some are able to say, "I'm not so good at team sports, so I do yoga," or "I have bad joints, so I prefer swimming." Some can even admit, "I just can't seem to make myself exercise. The only way I can make myself exercise is to do something that doesn't look like exercise." We can make exercise work better for us as we accept our weaknesses. Then, we can choose to work on and strengthen them. Doing so is part of embracing self-worth.

On the flip side, we must also accept our strengths. Acknowledging, "I'm really good at walking," or "getting myself out of bed to stretch in the morning," or "playing tag with my kids," helps us discover joy in exercise. Research shows that when we identify and use our signature strengths, we experience greater happiness and life satisfaction (Seligman, 2004).

Do This . . . Self-Acceptance

Return to your lists of strengths and weaknesses, above. Read each one out loud and ask yourself, "Do I accept this about myself?" Pay close attention to those qualities that you are unsure, anxious, or in any way uncomfortable about. These are likely traits you have yet to accept. Circle them, and then, using the ideas presented here, work on accepting them.

Self-Love

Practicing self-awareness and self-acceptance are helpful precursors to learning self-love—to loving who we really are and who we have the potential to become. It's not good enough to simply accept who and how we are. If we want to experience self-worth, we must learn to love who we are.

Self-love consists of four practices:

1. *Self-Kindness.* This involves doing kind and thoughtful things for yourself, such as letting yourself go out with your partner, calling a friend to catch up, grabbing some takeout after a long day, or even going for a hike on a gorgeous summer morning. Self-kindness helps us feel mentally and emotionally healthier because it gives us permission to recognize and meet our needs. Whatever you would do for someone else—to be kind, help, show thoughtfulness—do that for yourself. This includes giving yourself oppor-

tunities to develop and share your strengths, and weaknesses, so you can grow.

2. *Self-Compassion.* Instead of criticizing yourself when you don't go for your scheduled jog, be compassionate. Remind yourself that it's okay, you can make up for it tomorrow, and then let it go. Instead of judging yourself for poor fitness or mental health, use that energy to get out and go for a walk, talk with a friend, or see that counselor you've been thinking of. Be compassionate with yourself. (If this is a struggle for you, don't worry. We will work more on changing your thoughts and beliefs in Key 5.)

3. *Letting love in.* It's impossible to feel self-worth if we block, ignore, or refuse love. Loving ourselves opens us up to receive greater love from others, thus continuing the cycle of giving and receiving love. Next time someone offers you a compliment, say "thank you" and leave it at that. Receive a smile from a stranger. Let others help you get a break, or exercise. Ask for and receive help when you need it. You'll have so much more love in your heart if you simply let love in.

4. *Love your Higher Power.* Letting yourself embrace the love that is bigger and greater than us all is a fundamental element of self-worth. It is knowing we are worthy just because we are. It is knowing there is grace, support, and divine potential waiting, if we choose to look, see, and let it in.

Together, these things create self-worth, or the experience of being worthy, loveable, and possessing potential—the potential to make exercise work for you, reap its mental health and self-esteem benefits, and use exercise throughout your life to improve your life. The potential to fulfill your dreams, become the person you desire to be, and the potential to know that person is someone incredible.

Do This . . . Self-Love

Use your list of strengths and weaknesses, and your notes from the self-acceptance exercise above, to practice self-love. Select one strength and one weakness and apply at least one of the four elements of self-love. For instance, if you struggle to accept that you're a good leader, then you might create an opportunity to share your leadership skills by organizing a group exercise class. You'll get to help others and exercise, plus practice letting love in when your friends thank you. Do the same for one weakness on your list. When you feel more accepting of that one, choose another and continue working down the list.

A Few More Tools for Self-Worth

Remember Mechelle's story, from Key 1? When Mechelle's marriage ended, it felt like her life ended, too. The depression and pain she felt immobilized her, filling her with extremely negative beliefs and thoughts about herself and her situation. Reading her story, it's obvious that Mechelle's path back to self-worth, joy, and health was a long and painful one, but she chose to take that path and do the work, and eventually, those early morning running sessions became Mechelle's lifeline. They moved her forward, despite the pain in her heart. They gave her confidence, and helped her trust herself and believe.

When it comes to self-worth, we need to discover and feel it, then put what we've discovered into practice. In addition to continually working on the principles of The Pyramid of Self-Worth, the following tools can help you do as Mechelle did and practice what you seek.

Banish Negative Self-Talk

If you seek self-confidence and empowerment, then you need to identify and banish the negative self-talk that so often accompanies a poor sense of self-worth. As you become aware of, accept, and love yourself for who you really are, you'll find that the negative thoughts and feelings you once had will no longer apply. The trick is to hear and stop them, or change them into more positive, helpful, and loving self-talk. Key 5 outlines strategies for changing our mind and thinking, but for now, start listening for the negative messages and try to challenge or banish them when they come.

Grieve

Mechelle found that running helped her process and grieve the loss of her marriage. If you've experienced a significant loss—recently or in the past—and haven't dealt with it, it's time to do so, and as we'll see below, exercise can help. Unprocessed grief can contribute to mental health issues and disorders, and when it's locked up deep inside, can impact self-worth. Self-acceptance means we have to accept all aspects of ourselves—even painful loss and grief.

Often, we don't allow ourselves to grieve because we simply don't know how. That's a question I hear often when it comes to loss—"How do I grieve?" My answer has always been, "You just do." But, a few years ago, I created a model to help people work through the grief process, to show them what to do. It's called TEARS. TEARS stands for: Talking, Exercise or physical activity, Artistic expression and creativity, Recording and writing experiences and emotions, and Sobbing.

Talk about your losses. Tell as many loved ones and trusted friends as it takes to feel the pain release. Talk to a counselor, faith leader, or doctor, especially if you need additional support and tools for how to handle the grief. Just talk.

Exercise. This is, after all, an exercise book, but exercise was on this list long before I even knew I would write this book because it helps. Move your body. Lift weights or do push-ups to release the muscle tension of grief. Walk, bike, or climb to lift the depression or anger of grief. Play with your kids in the yard or on a team sport to lift your spirits. Just move.

Be **Artistic** and creative. Paint, write, sing, dance, draw, sculpt, mold, create. Use your creativity to process your loss. Create a collage of favorite memories of a lost loved one with your children. Dance out your grief over your divorce. I have lost many loved ones, and I've almost always written them a song after. It helps me process my feelings and express my love, which is what grieving is all about.

Record or write how you're feeling. Journal, write, type, scribble. Whatever helps you process what you're going through, do that. Then, you can revisit it later and better understand.

Sob. Cry, and let it all out. For as long as you need.

Believe You're Worth It

The biggest thing Mechelle gained through her experiences with exercise and healing was the knowledge that she was worth it. Those runs empowered Mechelle. They formed the truths that made her who she is today. "I am brave, strong and competent," she says now, and she is.

When it comes to exercise for mental health, often the biggest thing in our way is ourselves. We resist believing we are worth it—worth the time, the effort, the success. Well, let me tell you— "You are worth it!" You are worth the time away from your partner and kids. You are worth the effort it takes to plan and execute physical activity. You are worth greater mental health, and peace, and happiness.

You're worth it. Remind yourself of my words. Highlight them. Write them on a sticky note and post it on your mirror—"You're worth it!" Then, use the principles and tools from this key and the keys to come to prove it to yourself, to accept, and to believe it.

Reflection Questions: Self-Esteem and Self-Worth

1. Pay attention to your thoughts and beliefs—about yourself, exercise, and mental health. Do you ever hear neg-

ative self-talk? If so, what does it sound like? Write all that comes to you down, below. (We'll revisit these in Key 5.)

---

2. Are there losses in your life you have yet to grieve that may stand in the way of your exercise for mental health success? If so, please seek to identify them, write them down, and then use TEARS to begin the grief process. How might everyday losses like loss of safety, security, goals, plans, and yes, self-worth, impact your exercise and mental health?

---

3. Do you believe in yourself when it comes to exercise and mental health? Do you feel empowered? Why or why not? What types of self-messages empower you?

_____

_____

_____

_____

_____

4. Review the research and thoughts above on self-esteem. What do you think? Do you think the pursuit self-esteem is a myth? Do you ever find yourself caught up in your thoughts, feelings, behaviors, or other's opinions about you—or the pursuit of self-esteem? How does it affect your exercise routine or mental health? Write it down.

_____

_____

_____

_____

_____

_____

_____

_____

5. Write your thoughts on self-worth and The Pyramid of Self-Worth. Which seems hardest for you—self-awareness, self-acceptance, or self-love? Why? Write about it on the lines below or in your journal.

_____

_____

_____

_____

_____

_____

_____

_____

6. Continue to use the exercises above to work through The Pyramid of Self-Worth, or add your own ideas. Keep track of your progress by writing about it in your journal, on your electronic device, or below. (For more help with The Pyramid of Self-Worth, visit http://www.exercise4mental health.com.)

_____

_____

_____

_____

_____

_____

_____

_____

_____

_____

_____

_____

_____

_____

_____

_____

_____

_____

_____

KEY 3

EXERCISE AS A FAMILY

"To resist the frigidity of old age, one must combine the body, the mind, and the heart. And to keep these in parallel vigor, one must exercise, study, and love."

—Alan Bleasdale

We move now from the internal workings of building and embracing self-worth to the external influences our family can have on us—on our perceptions of who we are, how we feel about exercise, and the formation of our mental and emotional well-being.

Family plays one of the most critical roles in how we view ourselves—in how we think and feel about who we are, are perceived in this world, and our attitudes toward a host of things, not least of which includes physical activity. Family is also one of the biggest influencers of our mental health. Healthy family environments promote and strengthen mental health, while unhealthy family systems can provoke or contribute to mental illness. It's therefore no surprise that exercising as a family is one of the best "keys" for mental health and physical activity across the lifespan. When the family is able to create and foster a positive relationship with exercise and physical activity, the entire family benefits, both physically and mentally.

Mental Health and Family

Whether you're living full-time with family members, raising your own family, or somewhere in-between or beyond, your family plays a bigger role in your mental health and exercise than you probably realize. First, let's examine the facts on mental health in family members, including children, adolescents, and parents. Then, we'll take a closer look at how exercise impacts each group and learn strategies to improve family physical activity.

Childhood Mental Health

The physical and mental health benefits of exercise presented in Key 1 apply equally to children, and exercise also positively impacts the developing brain. Helping a child be active can significantly improve his mood, focus, self-esteem, and overall happiness. If we can get kids moving, we may not only be able to treat their mental health symptoms; we may also prevent mental illness, creating a lifelong habit of exercise for mental health.

Mental health disorders occur in children more commonly than most people think. Research shows that 15 million children are currently diagnosed with a mental health disorder, and even more children are at high risk for developing mental illness in the future due to genetic, family, school, social, and community stressors/factors (American Psychological Association [APA], 2015). In fact, childhood mental diagnoses are on the rise, with pediatricians identifying mental illness in only 8.1% of children in 2010 versus 10.5% in 2013, an increase of 29% (Sung, 2013). The most common childhood mental health issues, in order of prevalence, include: attention-deficit/hyperactivity disorder (ADHD), behavioral or conduct problems, anxiety disorders, depression, and autism-spectrum disorders (Perou et al., 2013).

Young children typically do not have the capacity to grasp what is going on with their mental or emotional health. The higher brain skills of insight and abstract thinking don't begin to develop until adolescence, and the brain isn't fully developed until about age 25. Because of this, and also because of the lack of control children have over their environment, care, and experiences, a child's mental health is weaved complexly with her physical health, school success, and family and social relationships.

Adolescent Mental Health

Adolescence presents a whole new set of challenges to mental health, and they primarily have one name: hormones. Hormone levels increase as children grow into adolescence, leading to the developing-body-and-mind phase of life we call puberty. Not only is the body changing, but also changes in hormones can wreak havoc on a young teen's brain by triggering emotional shifts, outbursts, and even mental illness.

Additionally, the teen years are a time of identity formation, with one of the biggest questions of life being, "Who am I?" As the brain develops and abstract and critical thinking emerge, adolescents begin to formulate their thoughts, beliefs, and experience of who they are in this world and how the world works. It's a crucial time in development, and thanks to increased pressure and stress in school, extracurriculars, or home life, it's also a vulnerable time for mental illness.

Depression risk actually increases as children move into adolescence and grow older, and it's estimated that 11% of teens have a depressive disorder by age 18 (NIMH, 2015a), and three of four people diagnosed with mental illness will show signs before age 24 (USDHHS, 2015). Yes, adolescence, and even early adulthood, can be a sensitive time, and untreated mental illness in young people can often develop into long-term mental illness.

Youth and Mental Health Treatment

Together, these facts demonstrate the need for education and early intervention to help children and teens navigate the tricky years when they're at high risk. Young people can receive effective treatment for mental health issues through psychotherapy, medication, or combined treatment, and the earlier in their illness they receive treatment, the more effective it will be (NIMH, 2009).

Unfortunately, only about 7% of children will receive the help they need (U.S. Public Health Service, 2000) and an estimated 60% of adolescents suffering from depression will receive no treatment at all (SAMHSA, 2014). While parents are likely to intervene if their child is getting drunk or using drugs, it's easy to overlook the teen who's watching too much TV, not participating in sports, or not sleeping enough. Additionally, parents may not understand the nature or severity of childhood or adolescent mental illness, and too often, it goes unnoticed and/or untreated.

Many parents and mental health providers are wary of medication in youth because of the side effects. They also show concern because their brains are still developing. Though in many cases medications are extremely helpful, it can be difficult to make the choice to medicate a child. Psychotherapy is a valuable resource for youth, especially when their parents or caregivers are willing to participate. Most schools have a counselor who may be able to provide free therapy. However, due to the stigma, time commitment, and financial concerns, many children are never taken to therapy. Sometimes those that are permitted to see a counselor have parents who do not wish to be involved.

Exercise is a valid alternative or addition to youth treatment options of all types. It's cost effective, safe, healthy, and it works on physical and mental health concerns. Helping children get out and move also combats too much screen time, which is associated with poorer mental health (Biddle & Asare, 2011). So much attention is focused on how exercise can fight obesity and keep kids physically healthy, and certainly that is important. However, it needs to be said, and said clearly: increasing exercise and physical activity in children and adolescents is one of the single best things we can do to reduce and prevent childhood mental illness and increase overall mental health and life satisfaction.

Parental Mental Health

Parents are also at risk for mental health concerns, starting with pregnancy, but continuing beyond.

It's estimated that one in five women will experience postpartum depression, 15% will experience pregnancy depression, and as many as 6% of pregnant and 10% of postpartum women will experience some form of anxiety disorder, including panic disorder, OCD, or PTSD. These disorders represent a spectrum of mental health concerns called perinatal mood and anxiety disorders. They are real and affect more mothers than most of us realize, pointing to the stress and vulnerability of the childbearing experience on mental well-being. In fact, a woman is 30 times more likely to experience a psychotic episode in the days following childbirth than any other time in her life, and one in 1,000 new mothers will experience postpartum psychosis, a serious and potentially life-threatening disorder that requires immediate treatment to protect both the mother and the baby.

Dads can also experience postpartum depression. It's estimated that as many as 10% of fathers worldwide and 14% in the United States experience paternal postnatal depression, or PPND (Paulson, 2010). And when one parent is depressed, there's a 50% chance the other parent will be, too. This can place a tremendous strain on the couple's relationship, and the first year postpartum has often been quoted as having the highest rates of divorce/separation than any other time in a couple's life (Arizona Postpartum Wellness Coalition, 2005).

Stress and lack of sleep are also common in adults, especially in parents. The relationship goes both ways: lack of sleep contributes to stress, and stress contributes to lack of sleep, both of which can have detrimental physical and mental health consequences. Sleep deprivation may start postpartum and last for months, or years, contributing to serious physical and mental health issues. Insomnia can cause problems well into middle adulthood as the busyness of work and family life seems to be never-ending. In addition to work and personal responsibilities, parents have added responsibility of caregiving, providing for, spending time with, and teaching their families. Even adults with no children are likely to experience caregiving for aging parents or family members in middle age, all of which can create significant stress.

In mid-life, perimenopause can be a significant contributor to mental health issues for women, as the menstrual cycle begins to slow and diminish. This phase of life often brings physical and emotional symptoms that can severely disturb a woman's mental health and, similar to the childbearing years, can present a huge strain on relationships.

For men, "mid-life crisis" is common, and can lead to higher rates of heavy drinking and even suicide in middle-aged men (Doheny, 2008), also creating problems for couples and family relationships.

Overall, family members may each present with their own unique vulnerabilities to mental illness. Considering the plethora of benefits exercise brings to the table, it seems the logical solution for improved family mental health.

Physical Activity and the Family

Unfortunately, most families do not engage in regular exercise.

Children, Teens, and Physical Activity

Kids are drastically failing to meet current standards for physical activity. A survey of 39 states by the National Institute of Health examined the activity levels, eating habits, emotional health, body image, and life satisfaction of nearly 10,000 students, ages 11 to 16, and found that only half of American adolescents are physically active five or more days a week, and less than one in three eat fruits and vegetables. Overall, they reported that 74% of youth do not live a healthy lifestyle (Iannotti & Wang, 2013).

Another interesting element of this study was that the researchers established three different categories of youth: healthful (27%), unhealthful (26%), and typical (47%). They found that "typical" youth were more likely than the other two groups to be overweight/ obese and to report greater body dissatisfaction. The unhealthful youth were more likely to be undernourished/underweight, to engage in the most screen time (TV, video games, and using the computer), and also reported the highest levels of depression and lowest levels of life satisfaction. The healthful adolescents, most of whom exercised five or more days a week, were the least likely to eat sweets and spend time in front of a screen, and reported the lowest rates of depression and highest life satisfaction ratings. Overall, however, this study reported that all groups could stand to improve their health and activity habits (Iannotti & Wang, 2013). The most discouraging finding of this large-scale study is that the majority of American children are losing a positive sense of body image and life satisfaction (Olson, 2013).

The American Heart Association (AHA) recommends that all children 2 years old and older should engage in "at least 60 minutes of enjoyable, moderate-intensity physical activities every day that are developmentally appropriate and varied" (2014). Yes, children as young as 2 should be enjoying regular physical activity. Yet, only one in three children is physically active each day and, on average, children now spend more than seven-and-one-half hours a day in front of a screen (President's Council on Fitness, Sports, & Nutrition, 2015). Teens are falling even farther behind, with an estimated 80% failing to get enough daily activity (USDHHS, 2015).

This is not just a problem for youth.

Adults and Physical Activity

Exercise is a valuable preventative and treatment option for mental health in the childbearing years, middle age, and beyond. Research has shown exercise can significantly elevate mood in pregnant and postpartum women, and men, and should be considered a first-line treatment option, especially since so many mothers worry about the risks of antidepressant use (Daly, Macarthur, & Winter, 2007). Exercise is not only safe for moms and dads; it's safe for babies and children. Exercise also promotes physical and mental health in pregnancy, postpartum, and parenting. It's truly a win-win.

Many parents and adults do not exercise, however.

- It's estimated that less than 5% of adults engage in the recommended 30 minutes of physical activity each day (U.S. Department of Agriculture [USDA], 2010), and only one in three adults obtain the recommended amount of exercise each week (USD-HHS, 2010).
- Only 28-34% of adults ages 65 to 74 and 35-44% of those 75 years and older are physically active (CDC, 2011).
- Overall, more than 80% of adults fail to meet the recommended levels of both aerobic and strength-training exercise (USDHHS, 2015).

There are many reasons adults fail to exercise. For parents, having a child often shifts priorities from oneself to one's child. While this can no doubt be a good thing, many parents give up their own physical and mental fitness as a result. Some feel, with such a full life, physical activity is no longer as important as it once was. Of course, lack of sleep can also impact motivation and ability to exercise, as well as the heavy responsibilities new parents face. Finally, having a baby or young children can make it tough for many parents to find the time and space to exercise.

Studies have shown that dating and marriage don't seem to impact exercise levels, but having a child most definitely reduces physical activity in adults. One study found that having a child decreased physical activity by three hours per week, with 66% of those with children falling below the average physical activity levels of their same-age, childless counterparts (Hull et al., 2010). For adults of all life phases, time and stress are two major barriers to physical activity. Thus, a family-centered approach is often ideal. Combining exercise with family time not only saves time, it's also a wonderful stress-reliever and helps families bond.

These are just a few of the many reasons to turn to family-based exercise for a solution: it's good for parents, good for kids, and a great way to build stronger families.

The Family Who Exercises Together . . .

Exercise isn't just for twenty-somethings. It's not just for athletic, coordinated people. Exercise is not just about losing weight, and it's not just for a certain period of life. Exercise is beneficial throughout the lifespan, with unique gifts for every season life brings, and as we look at the influence the family has on exercise across the lifespan, it's easy to see that exercising as a family is one of the most valuable habits we can establish for a lifelong love of exercise and optimal mental health.

Having a supportive family, and friends, has consistently been shown in the research to be one of the strongest predictors of increased exercise and activity in youth (Duncan, Duncan, & Strycker, 2005), developing in young people a habit of health and activity that continues well into adulthood. The same goes for all other members of the family. Family-based interventions and approaches to physical activity have the potential to instill the values and beliefs about exercise that keep us exercising for life (Brustad, 2010).

There are myriad ways we might finish the sentence, "The family that exercises together . . ." Exercising as a family benefits not only the individual family members, but also the family system as a whole, and in a variety of ways. Let's take a look at what the research has to say.

The family that exercises together:

. . . gets, and stays, healthy together— physically and mentally

In Key 1, we explored the research on how exercise can benefit your mental health. Now, imagine that your entire family can receive those benefits. The truth is, they can.

All of the physical health benefits of exercise we outlined in Key 1 can also apply to the children, adolescents, and adults (of any age) in your family. Exercise is important for families because it can lower heart risks, control weight, improve school performance, and increase life expectancy (Bhargava, 2014). Additionally, all of the mental health benefits outlined in Key 1 can apply to each of your family members. Family exercise can improve mental and emotional well-being, reduce stress and anxiety, and improve happiness and overall life satisfaction for everyone, creating a happier, healthier family unit.

One interesting study examined the progress of recovering stroke patients who were randomly assigned to either the control group, who received routine therapy including exercise, or the family-based group, who received routine therapy and a family-mediated exercise program where family members were responsible for providing structured, quantifiable activity each day. Results showed that the family-based exercise program not only led to increased confidence and a more positive experience in the stroke patients, but the caregivers in this group reported significantly lower levels of caregiver strain compared to their control group counterparts, empowering them with the skills they needed to help their loved ones (Galvin et al., 2011).

This is just one of many examples of how exercising as a family benefits all family members, and in powerful ways. Incorporating not just physical health (i.e. improved nutrition and diet) but also mental health-promoting education and practices, along with exercise will result in healthier, happier, and more satisfied families.

. . . grows in self-worth and confidence together

In Key 2 we discussed how exercise makes us feel better about ourselves and can lead to a greater sense of self-worth. One proposed theory for how this happens is called self-determination theory. Self-determination theory proposes that we feel motivated to engage in physical activity when: 1) we feel competent at it, 2) we feel we can exert personal control during the activity, and 3) we feel a strong connection with others while engaging in the activity.

Research indicates that children will be more likely to engage in physical activity and to perceive it as "fun" when they feel competent in that activity (Brustad, 2010), and let's face it—adults feel the same way. We like doing activities we're good at; we enjoy them more when we feel competent. This sense of competency and confidence in physical activity has been shown to affect our lifelong exercise habits and practices (Brustad, 2010). This is a significant point for families to comprehend, since family support is one of the best ways to bolster a child's sense of personal control and self-efficacy in physical activities (Dzewaltowski et al., 2010), and these children are then more likely to grow into adults who value and practice exercise. Put plainly, children (and adults) are much more likely to want to exercise, and keep exercising, when they feel intrinsically motivated—when they feel confident, a sense of control, and connected to others during the activity. The family is an ideal place to develop that motivation.

We first learn self-worth and confidence in the home. If we want our children and spouse/partner to develop a habit of exercise for mental health for life, we should also try to demonstrate self-worth and confidence. As we provide our family members with opportunities to be active and try new activities, encourage and guide one another in learning new exercise skills, work together, and yes, have fun, we will grow together in confidence and self-worth. (We'll discuss self-determination theory and motivation more in Key 4).

. . . has fun together

Exercise is not only good for our body and mind; it's good for the soul—if we do it right. Exercise and activity can, and should, be fun. It should involve play, laughter, and memory making with family and friends. Kids are all about having fun, and games, sports, and activities like jumping rope, playing tag, and doing tricks on the trampoline are fun—and great exercise.

But the fun isn't just for the kids. Parents who make exercise fun for kids benefit by having a little fun, too. Family bike rides, hikes, walks at sunset, family soccer games, or even just heading off in the woods to explore, allow families to smile, laugh, and make memories together, and it doesn't usually feel like exercise. That's the great part. Kids don't necessarily care that exercise will help them burn off energy, keep their minds fresh, promote their mental and physical health, and create healthy habits that will last a lifetime. When we find ways to make exercise feel like play, the entire family is more likely to learn to enjoy exercising, and to stay with it long-term (Bhargava, 2014).

. . . remains active together, throughout life

It's no question that parental support and example is one of the biggest factors in those who become, and stay, active throughout their lives. Research shows that physical activity "tracks" from childhood through adolescence and into adulthood, meaning that active children tend to be active adolescents who tend to be active adults (Brustad, 1993; Pate et al., 1996).

The family plays a principal role in this. Active parents tend to have active children. One study of 4- to 7-year-olds found that children with two active parents were nearly six times more likely to be active, too. Even more interestingly, they found that children with one active and one inactive parent were still more than three times more likely to be active than children with two inactive parents (Moore et al., 1991). Additional research has shown significant relationships between the physical activity levels of every possible family member combination (i.e. mother-father, father-son, mother-daughter, siblings, and so on) (Seabra et al., 2008), providing even greater evidence that families who are active together tend to stay active, together.

. . . stays together

Exercising as a family doesn't just create physically and mentally healthy individuals, though that is a huge payoff. It creates a healthier family unit. Being active together doesn't just help wear kids out so they'll go to bed earlier and sleep longer (which, let's face it parents, is a bonus). No. Exercise has the potential to bring families closer.

Think about it. If your family can get out and walk, ride, climb, swim, skip, hop, run, jump, play, and explore together, you'll be creating lifelong health habits with the added bonus of the quality togetherness most time-starved families desperately need today (Trost & Loprinzi, 2011). Exercising as a family promotes bonding, creates memories, strengthens family members, and fortifies the family as a whole. What could be better than that?

The Impact of Family on Exercise and Mental Health Attitudes, Beliefs, and Values

Hopefully, you're feeling inspired to get your family moving, but first, it's important to emphasize the connection between exercise and mental health attitudes with our beliefs and values, and our family of origin.

Our family's values, beliefs and attitudes about mental health and physical activity most certainly shape our own (Brustad, 2010). Children tend to rely upon parents for feedback and judgment as they strive to form their own beliefs about their competence, likes and dislikes, and attitudes about physical activity and mental health (Brustad, 2010). In most cases, our first beliefs and values come directly from our parents and our family, and children tend to form pretty stable attitudes and beliefs about physical activity and exercise by early elementary school (Brustad, 1993; Rose et al., 2009). These beliefs typically apply to other ideas and practices as well, like appropriate nutrition and diet, attitudes about mental illness, and beliefs about mental, emotional, social, and spiritual health, all of which are most typically learned and reinforced in the family context.

We just discussed how family members tend to be similar in their activity levels, and it should come as no surprise, then, that family members are also similar in their attitudes and beliefs about physical activity. This makes sense, doesn't it, since the family is where we, as children, are first exposed to various forms of physical activity and the beliefs around it. When we are raised in a home that either doesn't value or devalues exercise, we will most likely struggle to value it ourselves. Parents are considered the gatekeepers of children's activity, either enabling or restricting opportunities to get out and move, and parents' beliefs, attitudes, and practices around physical activity are some of the strongest predictors of the behaviors and beliefs of their children (Brustad, 2010).

This doesn't mean we can't change the beliefs and attitudes handed down by our parents. Not at all. It simply means that if we don't make ourselves aware of the family values and attitudes that might stand in our way, it can make it harder for us to value exercise for mental health. Many of us may not have even noticed that we've adopted our family's beliefs and attitudes about mental health and exercise as our own, nor see how those beliefs are standing in our way. Until we understand the values and beliefs behind our own attitudes about mental health and exercise, we'll remain unable to move past them.

So, pull out a pen or pencil, find a quiet space, and give yourself a few minutes to honestly answer the following questions about your family of origin's attitudes, beliefs, values, and practices. Then, give yourself time to reflect upon how these things might influence your own attitudes, values, beliefs, and practices about exercise for mental health.

Reflection Questions: Family of Origin

1. How active would you say your family of origin was when you were growing up, on a scale of 1-5? (1=completely inactive; 5=highly active) Would you say you're similar or different from your family of origin's activity level? Why?

_____

_____

_____

_____

_____

_____

2. What messages, ideas, or beliefs did/does your family put forth about exercise and physical activity?

_____

_____

_____

_____

_____

_____

_____

3. What beliefs or values did/does your family put forth about mental illness, mental health, and the treatment or prevention of such conditions?

_____

_____

_____

_____

_____

_____

_____

4. How might each of these family values have impacted your own values and beliefs surrounding exercise and mental health?

_____

_____

_____

5. Did you feel competent in physical activity as a child? In what ways do you think your family influenced your level of self-confidence in physical activity? Did they support and build your confidence? Did they minimize or prevent you from developing exercise self-confidence? Or, were they indifferent when it came to supporting and encouraging you in physical activity? How do you feel about this, and how confident do you feel about physical activity today?

_____

_____

_____

_____

_____

_____

_____

_____

_____

_____

_____

_____

_____

Challenges to Family Exercise

Beliefs and attitudes aren't the only blocks to family exercise. It can be tough to get everyone on board, and for a variety of reasons.

With kids, some of the common challenges include:

- *Kids don't think exercise is fun.* This is probably one of the biggest reasons kids aren't more active. But we're going to change that.
- *They prefer doing other, more sedentary, activities.* Watching TV, playing video games, or going on the computer is way more appealing that getting up and moving for many kids.
- *Some feel embarrassed trying exercise for the first time.* When they don't know what to do, as we discussed above, it can kill their confidence and stop exercise before it even begins.
- *They try but feel exercise is uncomfortable or hard to do.* It can feel this way for all of us when we're just starting, but there are ways to overcome this, as we'll see below.

Teens face some unique challenges that can make it difficult for them to want to engage in exercise, as well:

- *They're "too busy" to exercise.* Between homework, social events, activities, and family responsibilities, teens are busy. It can be tough for them to want to add an extra thing to their full lifestyle.
- *They're too tired.* Teens are tired—too tired, usually. They actually need more sleep than parents realize, especially since their brains and bodies are undergoing such a complete overhaul.
- *They're strong-willed.* The developing adolescent brain can make teens more strong-willed and opinionated about what they want or are willing to do. They may simply not want to exercise, and it can be tough for parents to get them to do so.
- *They "have a life."* Time with friends is tops in the teen's mind. If exercise is interfering with their social life, it's not going to fly.

Truth be told, all of these challenges, for teens and for kids, apply to adults and parents, as well. We don't always think exercise is fun, we'd rather be doing other things, and we may feel embarrassed or uncomfortable when we're exercising for the first time. We're busy, tired, sometimes strong-willed, and yes, we want to "have a life," too. There are plenty of reasons not to exercise, and it's important to identify those that apply most to you if you want to overcome them. Key 6 is all about overcoming the roadblocks to exercise, but right now, let's take a moment to examine what some of your family's roadblocks might be.

Reflection Questions: Family Roadblocks

1. Go back and re-read the "challenges to exercise" above. Which of these seem to be your biggest personal roadblocks? Which seem to block your family's exercise for mental health potential?

_____

_____

_____

_____

_____

_____

_____

_____

2. What personal challenges do you face when it comes to being physically active?

_____

_____

_____

_____

_____

_____

3. What challenges do your children, spouse/partner, and family face that make exercise for mental health difficult?

_____

_____

_____

_____

_____

_____

_____

_____

4. What do you feel your family most needs to help you overcome these roadblocks?

_____

_____

_____

_____

Creating Healthy Family Attitudes, Values, and Beliefs about Exercise and Mental Health

If we want ourselves, and our families, to grow to value exercise, then "promoting physical activity for children and youth in such a way that it will result in lifelong motivation and involvement is particularly important" (Brustad, 2010, p. 1). How do we do this? For starters, the younger we are taught the value physical activity, the more ingrained it becomes in who we are and the longer we're likely to stay with it. This doesn't mean that it's too late for adults, it's just that the sooner we begin prioritizing exercise, the better—for everyone. Here are some suggestions to get you started.

When it comes to family exercise, remember the following do's and don'ts.

Do This. . .

- *Focus on being active, not on "exercise."* You don't have to even use the word "exercise" if you don't want to. Just encourage your family to move—as much and as often as possible.
- *Focus on health—mental and physical—not on weight loss.* Your

goal is to increase your family's activity in order to increase their mental, physical, emotional, social, and spiritual health, not to encourage your family members to lose weight.

- *Prioritize physical activity for your own mental health and be the example.* If you get moving, your kids and family are more likely to follow.
- *Model healthy beliefs and values about exercise.* Remember, you don't only model the behavior of being physically active; you also model the beliefs, attitudes, and emotions about exercise, physical health, and mental health (Brustad, 2010). Your family is watching and listening, so be careful what you say.
- *Provide opportunities for your family to be active.* Encourage everyone to participate in sports and other programs, and set up family opportunities to increase physical activity.
- *Participate in activities alongside your children as often as possible.*
- *Support and encourage your family members.* This is crucial in helping everyone learn to value activity. It helps them feel competent and confident, and encouraging your family will feel good to you, too.
- *Make it fun!* There are dozens of great ideas for how to do this, below.
- *Educate your family on the benefits of exercise for mental health.* Teach kids how moving their bodies throughout the day can help them feel less stressed, more confident, and happier. (Just don't expect this to be a main motivator for them to exercise—you'll go a lot farther by using fun!)

Do . . .

- *Invite children of all ages to join you in your personal exercise.* Let your toddler stretch while you do yoga, put young kids in the stroller or let them ride a bike while you go for a jog. Invite teenagers to lift weights with you at the gym or at home.
- *Encourage your child to participate in and learn new sports, games, and activities.* Teach them the skills they'll need for these activities, to boost their confidence and sense of competency.

- *Set the example by engaging in and learning new sports, exercises, and activities.* Practice the new skills you learn in order to boost your own confidence and sense of competency and model this for your children.
- *Limit family screen time.* Too much time in front of the TV or video games is correlated with lower rates of activity and poorer mental health for everyone, so turn off the TV and get outside.
- *Involve friends and pets.* Getting together with friends or other families is great motivation, and pets (namely dogs) are, too. They need exercise and they'll force you out the door to do it.
- *Be an advocate for physical activity and sports programs in your community.* Encourage schools and communities to create low-cost programs that are not just for "the best athletes," and that promote activity, learning, and fun.
- Remember, you play an extremely important role in helping your child and your family establish healthy physical and mental health habits and beliefs, and your family plays a crucial role in helping you, too.

Don't . . .

- *Give up.* Exercising as a family can be challenging and it can take some time to find a system that works, but the payoff is worth it. So, stick with it. Keep trying new ideas, including some of those below or your own. Keep encouraging and supporting and loving one another as you seek to be active together.

Ideas for Fun Family Activities

Use one of these suggestions or one of your own. The possibilities are endless, so find what works for your family and do it. Here are some examples:

- Give children toys that encourage physical activity, like balls, kites, and jump ropes.

- Facilitate a safe walk to and from school a few times a week.
- Take the stairs instead of the elevator.
- Walk around the block after a meal.
- Make a new house rule: no sitting still during television commercials.
- Find time to spend together doing a fun activity: family park, swim, or sports day.
- Volunteer to help with afterschool physical activity programs or sports teams.
- Go golfing, horseback riding, or snowshoeing together.
- Play ultimate Frisbee. (This is a family favorite around our house.)
- Play family soccer, football, or baseball.
- Explore your neighborhood, looking for animals, flowers, plants, trees, and people that peak your interest.
- Play monkey-in-the-middle.
- Play tag or hide and seek.
- Play catch or toss a football around.
- Play basketball games like HORSE, "Knock-Out," or see who can shoot the most baskets in one minute.
- Climb a hill, mountain, or tree.
- Do family relay or wheelbarrow races, or play tug of war.
- Have a family wrestling or arm-wrestling match. (Just don't get too competitive!)
- Play Twister or Charades together.
- Go rollerblading, ice skating, skiing, or snowboarding.
- Take a family bike ride.
- Roll down a hill and then run back up.
- Go swimming, splash, and see who can swim the farthest underwater or tread water the longest.
- Have a water balloon fight or an egg toss contest with family teams.
- Play racquet sports like tennis, pickleball, Smashball, or racquetball together.
- Create an obstacle course, have a Hula-Hoop competition, or try double-dutch jump rope.

- Play family volleyball, badminton, balloon volleyball, or if you dare, dodgeball.
- Take your dog to the park and throw a ball or Frisbee around together.
- Play follow the leader, Mother May I, Red Light/Green Light, or hopscotch.
- Take a kayak, canoe, or river-rafting trip.
- Plant and take care of a garden or your yard.
- Travel, and explore the sights on foot (or bike).
- Head to the beach and go surfing, boogie boarding, paddleboarding, or just jump and play in the waves.
- Get adventurous and try cliff jumping, ziplining, or do an adventure course together.
- Go hiking, rock-climbing, or try an indoor climbing gym or rock wall.
- Dance! Sing, twirl, jump, spin, move, and groove together. Make up a dance routine or just turn on the music and let yourself go!
- Try family yoga, Tai Chi, or Pilates.
- Do an exercise video together. Challenge each other to push harder and do better.
- In the winter, shovel snow from the driveway and build a snowman, have a snowball fight, go sledding together, or make snow angels.
- Clean the house to music, or make it a race to see who can pick up the most things in each room.
- Practice doing cartwheels, summersaults, or other gymnastics together.
- Play an active video game together like Wii Fit or a dancing game.
- On rainy days, try skating in socks on a wood floor.
- Make a goal to play at every park in your town.
- Whenever possible, encourage your family to take the stairs. If you have stairs at home, make it a goal to go up and down at least 10 times a day.
- Train as a family for a charity walk, climb, or run.
- Celebrate special occasions—like birthdays or anniversaries—

with something active, such as a hike, a volleyball or soccer game, or playing Frisbee at the park.

- Walk instead of driving whenever you can. If you have to drive, find a spot at the far end of the parking lot and walk to where you're going. Race back to the car, being sure to look out for traffic.

- Plan active family gatherings (hiking, rafting, tag, relay races, dance party, skating, family sports activity, sledding, skiing, and so on). When my husband's family gets together, we have pickle-ball, basketball, whiffle ball, or trampoline trick competitions. It can get pretty intense.

- Turn yard work into fun (jump in the raked pile of leaves or shoveled snow, or turn on the music and sing as you work).

- Make a game of chores. We like to move room-to-room as a family and set the timer for two minutes in each room. Then, we see who can pick up the most items as we get the whole house done in no time flat.

- Sneak activity into other activities, like shopping at the mall (take the stairs and walk quickly between stores).

- Turn TV commercials into fitness breaks. March, do jumping jacks, twist, or dance together until the show starts again.

- Have a weekly family sports night. Invite friends or neighbors to participate once in a while, too.

- Use pedometers to keep track of family members' daily steps. Issue a challenge to see who can take the most steps each day/week.

Create Fun Family Goals or Challenges

Attempt to engage all your family members in a common goal: the goal to increase physical activity. Make it a family challenge, or a game, and make it fun.

Present your family with the list of activities above and let each family member take turns choosing your activity for the day or week. Get everyone involved in planning and executing your family goal, and remind family members they will have to report, and be held accountable, for their activities each week. Use the goal-setting strategies outlined in Key 4 to help you set specific, achievable goals your family will enjoy.

Give each family member a pedometer and challenge family members to walk an extra 1,000 or 2,000 steps each day. Get creative. Watch a movie together and march in place during the commercials. Take the dog for extra walks each day, or walk around the house while you're on a phone call. Encourage your family members to find creative ways to get their daily steps in, too.

Encourage your family to engage in active transportation. Nowadays, few children and teens and even fewer adults use active means of transportation (i.e. walking, biking, skateboarding) to get to school and work. Yet, one study shows that children who bike or walk to school tend to stay more active throughout the day, and we can assume the same would apply to adults (Fulton et al., 2006). Families can ride or walk together to school or work. Pick up kids on your bike after school, or, on the weekends, walk to the city bus stop, take a trip downtown, and explore (don't forget to stop for a treat).

Issue a family challenge to see who can be the first to achieve a Presidential Active Lifestyle Award by committing to physical activity five days a week, for six weeks. Adults and children can both receive the award, and it's a great way to encourage your family to participate in a common goal.

Tips for Making Family Exercise Work

It's not easy to change your family habits, but it can be done. Here are a few suggestions to make it a little easier.

Set Goals

Setting family-focused, achievable goals is a great place to start. We will talk more about goal-setting strategies in Key 4, but for now, focus on specific goals—for instance, instead of saying, "We will be more active each week," say, "We will go for a family walk, hike, or bike ride three days a week minimum."

Schedule Activities

We schedule work, school, and extracurricular activities, so why not schedule family physical activity? Use a family calendar to keep family members organized, and each week, add in specific activities and the days you will do them. This can help family members prioritize exercise each week. An online calendar like the one found at letsmove.gov titled Let's Move Healthy Family, is another great solution to family activity scheduling (Let's Move, 2015).

Be Flexible

Yes, things will come up. Yes, kids will get sick, work will run late, family members will forget or be too busy. The important thing is to plan for disruptions by being flexible. If you can't fit in your weekly family sports activity, then play an active video game together instead. If the weekdays get too full, then pack in activities on the weekends. Remember, your goal is to increase family activity and move, and there are plenty of ways to do this if you're flexible and patient.

A New Version of Health and Exercise: Julie's Story

Julie is 33-year-old wife and mother of three. She had been struggling with anxiety since she was a teen, working with different psychotherapists along the way, and all had recommended exercise. But it wasn't until she was recovering from postpartum OCD, with her fourth therapist, that she decided to give exercise a concerted try.

Julie had powerfully negative feelings about exercise, but she believed that if she just pushed herself, eventually exercise would be something she enjoyed. She joined a small gym for women and worked out in an intimate group setting, but while she enjoyed getting out and interacting with others, the actual exercising made her feel mentally and physically worse. It caused nausea and sometimes, vomiting, that led to extreme negative self-talk. *You don't know what you're doing. It's not worth it. You're overweight and lazy. You're not worth it.* These thoughts beat her up before and after every workout. Yet, despite these mental and physical beatings, Julie stuck it out for two long years, never experiencing any of the mental and physical "payoffs" of exercise she so desperately sought. Finally, she could take it no longer, and, figuring, *What's the point?* she quit the gym, and exercise.

It wasn't until Julie and I were working together, a couple years later, that she began to identify and explore these negative thoughts and self-talk, through CBT and thought records (which we will learn all about in Key 5). It wasn't until we began to explore her family of origin's beliefs and attitudes toward exercise that the picture became clear.

Julie explained she lumped exercise into the category of "being healthy"—eating good foods, taking vitamins, and exercise all went together. Because of difficult circumstances between her parents, Julie had lived with her grandmother for a few years in childhood, and this grandmother, Julie says, was "mentally ill in her own way and was seriously OCD about being healthy." Julie was named after her aunt Julie, her grandmother's daughter, who passed away when she was thirteen months old from pneumonia and flu. "My grandma was against medical interventions and was into all things natural, so she refused medical treatment for her daughter," Julie says. "It was 1961. I don't doubt she'd be in prison had this happened in our day." Julie says, "My grandmother fed me things called broccoli patties. Gag me. Eggplant pizza was a treat. We had carob instead of chocolate." She was also given enemas to cleanse her body of illness. "It was so traumatizing for me," Julie says. Her grandmother also loved to exercise. "She kept a small trampoline and weights in her room and would walk miles a day, well into her nineties."

Julie's family's beliefs and expectations toward exercise and health were obviously high, but they weren't positive, especially not for Julie. "It was all unhealthy, in my opinion," she said, and to make things worse, mental illness was not acceptable in Julie's family either. "The belief was that if you ate healthy and exercised, you shouldn't have any problems, and if you were depressed, well it definitely wasn't something you should talk about with others."

As Julie and I explored these things, it became clear why Julie had such a powerful negative reaction to exercise and toward her grandmother's concept of "being healthy." Such extreme views and behaviors created in Julie an aversion. "I ran the opposite direction. Actually, I don't run. I eat junk. I don't exercise. I'm on my sixth therapist. I tell anyone that wants to listen about my struggles with mental illness. Sometimes, I over share." Understanding more about her family of origin helped Julie begin to heal.

First, Julie needed to be shown her strengths. She is obviously a highly dedicated and persistent person. She forced herself to exercise for two years, even though it made her physically sick and miserable. She has taken charge of her mental health by seeking help, being open, and even by sometimes sharing her struggles in public forums that touch and help other people. Julie is also a dedicated, loving mother. She not only cares for her own three children, but largely raised her two youngest siblings and recently became a foster mother to a newborn.

Next, Julie needed to reframe the concepts of "exercise" and "being healthy." It makes sense, knowing her family history, why Julie would reject anything that resembles her grandmother's version of health. She's right—it wasn't healthy. Any extreme is unhealthy. And that's what Julie needed help with. In her efforts to avoid her grandmother's beliefs and ways, Julie pushed to the opposite extreme, like a pendulum. She forgot there are all sorts of ways to be mentally and physically healthy, and exercise, that aren't at either extreme. She needed to settle somewhere in the middle.

Julie began to create her own version of "healthy" and "exercise," one that actually helped her. She began to see that moving her body makes her happy when she can do things that don't feel like "exercise." She loves to dance, with her kids and alone, and she'll blast a favorite song on repeat and make up a routine. It gets her heart rate up higher than the gym did, but she finds it so fun that she doesn't mind the discomfort. She counts trips to Costco as exercise, especially when toting a baby carrier and shopping for a family of six. Most recently, Julie's family has started walking together. She and her husband push the foster baby in a stroller while her kids ride bikes. "I love our neighborhood! It is great for walking," Julie has realized. "That is something I know I can do."

Though Julie still struggles to get up and move, she's beginning to see the light at the end of the tunnel. As she's begun to put the pieces to her exercise puzzle together, she's learning the power of family—for worse, or for better. As she involves her family in her new version of "health" and "exercise," and continues to challenge her thinking using the principles of CBT that we'll discuss in Key 5, Julie is finally able to overcome some of that negative self-talk. "Bottom line: I have to find what works for me and do it," Julie says. "I have to throw out my perception and beliefs of what exercise should be and find what I can be capable of maintaining long term." She is finding a way to create a healthier version of exercise and mental health than the one she grew up with, and it is paying off—for herself and her family.

Reflection Questions: Family Exercise

1. Consider your current season of life. What specific challenges do you face? What tips can you take away to help you overcome your specific life challenges? Write them down.

_____

_____

_____

_____

_____

_____

2. What benefits most interest you when it comes to family exercise? Review the lists of benefits and facts above and then write about those that matter most to you. How

might these things keep you motivated to continually seek to be active as a family?

_____

_____

_____

_____

_____

_____

_____

_____

_____

_____

_____

PART 2

Prepare

KEY 4

GET MOTIVATED

"Strength does not come from physical capacity. It comes from an indomitable will."

—Mahatma Gandhi

In Part 1, we outlined the numerous benefits of exercise on physical and mental health, self-esteem, and self-worth, and even on the family. Yet, research estimates that 50% of those who start an exercise program will drop out within the first six months (Wilson & Brookfield, 2009), and many may never even begin. If exercise is so clearly beneficial, then why is it such a challenge for most of us to stick with it? The answer begins with one concept: motivation.

What is Motivation?

We can all relate to feeling either motivated or unmotivated to do something, can't we? The first example that comes to mind is school and homework. I'm sure each of us can recall a time from school or college days when we needed to complete a paper, project, or studying, but we just didn't feel motivated to do it. Perhaps we were able to make ourselves get up and do it anyway, but perhaps we procrastinated and paid the price later. Either way, we know what motivation, or lack of motivation, feels like.

What we may not fully understand is what motivation really is, and how it really works. Motivation is a psychological construct used to explain behavior. It also helps us understand our desires, needs, wants, thoughts, and feelings. It's what gets us up and doing what we know we could, should, or need to do. It's what makes us want to change, grow, and improve. It explains why we want to repeat or to stop a behavior, and also helps us understand why we don't act—why we avoid, reject, or even fear certain behaviors, feelings, and experiences. Motivation is a word that's part of our daily thought process and vocabulary, and it's one of the most popular concepts that we've adapted from psychology into everyday life. Motivation is quite literally in everything we do (or don't do).

Unfortunately, for the most part, we don't understand or comprehend our own motivations. This is where so many of us get stuck. We know when we feel motivated. We know when we don't feel motivated. But how regularly do we check in, evaluate, and try to *understand* our motivations—our motivations for how we treat people, why we do the things we do, what we avoid, and yes, our motivations for our daily behaviors, including exercise? For most of us, I'd say, it's pretty infrequent.

The truth is we don't always know why we do what we do, and until we can understand our motivation, we'll continually struggle to get to where we want to be. Let's do an exercise to help illustrate what I mean. Please grab a pencil, find a quiet spot, and take a few moments to honestly ask yourself the following questions.

Reflection Questions: Self-Motivations

1. Why did I select this book to read in the first place? What motivated me to pick it up, and then to purchase or borrow it?

_____

_____

_____

_____

_____

_____

2. Once I had the book, what motivated me to open it and start reading?

_____

_____

_____

_____

_____

_____

3. What is currently motivating me to read about this particular key, on motivation? What do I hope to gain from reading this?

_____

_____

_____

_____

_____

_____

Did you answer the reflection questions? If so, what motivated you to take the time to do this exercise? Was it because I asked nicely? (I did say, 'please.') If you did not answer the reflection questions, then what motivated you to skip it?

See? Motivation is in everything that we do (or don't do), and when we begin to examine our motivations, we begin to find the key to initiative, drive, follow through, and ultimately, to achieving what we most desire.

Motivation to Begin Exercising

Starting physical activity can be the hardest part for many of us, and there are several reasons why, not least of which is our self-perception (we'll discuss overcoming other roadblocks in Key 6). The way we view ourselves (including our past experiences and present reality) directly impacts whether or not we will initiate an exercise program. Negative self-perceptions can even prevent people who desperately need exercise, for serious medical reasons, from exercising. Feeling incompetent, insecure, or even inexperienced in physical activity—in general or in specific physical activities—can prevent those who've never attempted to be active from trying. As we discussed in Key 3, feeling competent is a powerful influencer of whether or not we will try and whether or not we will keep trying.

Another aspect of self-perception involves future hopes. If we hope that in the future we'll feel physically and mentally healthy, be active, mobile, happy, and well, then we're more likely to start exercising now to obtain that future vision.

What creates the healthy self-perceptions that motivate us to begin exercise? Research consistently shows that we are more likely to initiate an exercise program when we receive: 1) positive feedback from family, friends, and fitness professionals, 2) reinforcement that exercise is beneficial and worthwhile, and 3) social support from loved ones. These three factors bolster our exercise-related self-perceptions and lead to greater motivation to start, and to continue, exercising (Whaley & Schrider, 2005).

Reflection Questions: Self-Perceptions

1. When it comes to exercise, how do I currently perceive myself? Do I believe I'm capable of exercising? Do I believe I'm competent? Do I feel self-confident? What self-perceptions do I hold that might impact my motivation to exercise?

_____

_____

_____

_____

_____

_____
_____
_____
_____

2. Where do I see myself in five years? Ten? Twenty? Do I see myself feeling physically active and mentally healthy? If so, why? If not, then why not?

_____
_____
_____
_____
_____
_____
_____
_____

3. How might my vision for my future play a role in my motivation to start exercising today?

_____
_____
_____
_____
_____
_____

Motivation to Keep Exercising

What motivates us to _keep_ exercising? It's more complex than we might think. A systematic review of the research by Stewart Trost and his colleagues (2002) found five major factors that influence exercise adherence:

1. **Demographic and biological factors.** Factors such as gender, age, and health are correlated with exercise adherence. Overall,

men, younger adults, and healthier individuals are more likely than women, older adults, and unhealthy individuals to continue physical activity (Trost et al., 2002).

2. **Psychological, cognitive, and emotional factors.** Self-efficacy, or the belief that we can effectively achieve a desired outcome, is considered one of the most important factors in exercise adherence, and sense of self-worth goes right along with it. Those who experience greater self-doubt, negative self-thinking, and insecurity are more likely to quit exercise (Huberty et al., 2008), while those who feel confident and successful at exercise are more likely to stay with it, long-term. Self-worth involves believing we are worth the time and effort it takes to exercise, and those who value themselves tend to exercise more. Women are more likely to struggle in this area. One's expectations of exercise can also work either for or against his ability to maintain exercise (Whaley & Schrider, 2005). For example, if I expect to feel calm and less stressed after going for a walk, but instead feel anxiety because of my accelerated heart rate, then I am more likely to quit exercising. (We'll discuss expectations in more detail, below.)

3. **Behavioral qualities and skills.** Research shows that those who seek a higher quality of life and prioritize exercise in their schedule tend to be the most consistent exercisers (Huberty et al., 2008). Additionally, those who understand the fitness and mental health gains of exercise and use this knowledge to improve their skills and competency are more likely to stick with it. Finally, when we enjoy how exercise improves our quality of life, when we feel and believe exercise truly benefits us in numerous ways, it can be a major motivator in helping us continue regular physical activity.

4. **Socio-cultural influences.** Social support from family and friends is highly important in keeping us motivated to exercise, and cultural support is just as vital. Culture can significantly impact how we exercise, how accepted we feel when we exercise, and our beliefs and values about exercise. Studies show that ethnic minority women have lower exercise adherence than white women (Allen & Morey, 2010) and several studies show the

important impact of social and economic issues on underserved and minority populations in their ability to access and adhere to exercise. When we approach exercise motivation with a social and cultural lens, we begin to see how different motivators may benefit different cultures and people. For example, research shows that for African American and Latino groups, both of whom tend to highly value family and community, incorporating friends and family into exercise leads to higher levels of exercise adherence (Orzech et al., 2013).

5. **Environment and physical activity characteristics.** Factors such as how available physical activity options are, transportation to and from sports and activities, and even concerns like safety and weather can significantly impact our motivation to exercise (Orzech et al., 2013). We're also influenced by how satisfied we feel with the activity itself, the fitness professionals, and exercise facilities available to us (Trost et al., 2002).

Exercise and Motivation: Self-Evaluation

This is why exercise motivation can seem so complex: many different factors play a role. And what the research has found is that regular self-evaluation is one of the best ways to identify and overcome the barriers and factors that interfere with exercise motivation. Self-assessment, evaluation, and even feedback from fitness professionals or trusted loved ones can be highly beneficial. Feedback can help us learn, develop skills, and make changes that keep us motivated. Positive feedback can help us believe in ourselves, feel confident, and set progressively more challenging goals, if we desire, to keep us growing (Whaley & Schrider, 2005).

Below is what I call an "Exercise Motivation Self-Evaluation." Please take some time to complete the questions, ponder, reflect, and honestly answer. We will revisit this evaluation later to help us in overcoming your specific motivational challenges to exercise for mental health.

Do This . . . Exercise Motivation Self-Evaluation

Complete the attached self-evaluation, or visit http://www
.exercise4mentalhealth.com to download a copy.

Exercise Motivation Self-Evaluation

How powerful is each of the following factors in motivating
or un-motivating you to exercise?
Next to each number, rate each factor from 0-5.
0=doesn't influence me at all; 1= influences me strongly for the
worse; 2=influences me for the worse; 3=sometimes for the worse,
sometimes for the better; 4=influences me for the better; 5=influ-
ences me strongly for the better.
You may circle more than one, as needed.

Demographic/Biological
    1. Age
    2. Gender
    3. Illness or health conditions
    4. Physical shape

Psychological/Cognitive/Emotional
    5. Current state of mental health
    6. Emotions/moods
    7. Life stress
    8. Insecurity
    9. Feeling good about myself
    10. Wanting to feel happier
    11. Overcoming mental illness
    12. Wanting to feel calmer
    13. Desire for greater mental clarity
    14. Desire to increase creativity
    15. Wanting to feel more relaxed
    16. Worries
    17. Fear of failure

18. Wanting to get/stay off medications
19. Fear of ridicule
20. Spirituality
21. Desire to sleep better
22. Eating habits
23. Feeling competent at exercise
24. Expectations of exercise
25. How I feel after I exercise
26. Negative self-talk/thinking
27. Desire for happiness
28. Impact on mental health

Behavioral/Body/Lifestyle

29. Poor planning/scheduling of exercise
30. Priorities
31. Laziness
32. Perfectionism
33. Kids/family responsibilities
34. My enjoyment of exercise (fun)
35. Lack of sleep/fatigue
36. Busyness
37. Work
38. Smoking, drugs, alcohol
39. Impact of exercise on my quality of life
40. Being physically healthier now
41. Being in shape
42. Long-term health gains
43. Overcoming bad habits
44. Losing weight
45. Long-term behavioral improvements
46. Being "thinner"
47. Increasing muscle mass
48. Being mentally healthier
49. Knowing the physical benefits of exercise
50. Knowing the mental health benefits of exercise
51. Being "buff" or "ripped"

52. Personal beliefs/values
53. My attitude
54. Feeling bored by exercise
55. Time it takes to exercise
56. Injury or soreness
57. Physical distress from exercise
58. External rewards (music, food, social connection, and so on)
59. Accountability to others

Socio-Cultural/Environmental

60. Family of origin beliefs/attitudes
61. Current family's attitudes/beliefs
62. Cultural norms/acceptance
63. Making friends
64. Support from family/friends
65. Financial issues
66. Exercise accessibility
67. Desire to strengthen relationships
68. Transportation to exercise
69. Weather
70. Satisfaction with exercise facilities/programs/professionals
71. Desire for social connection
72. Social pressures or distress
73. Safety concerns
74. Desire to live longer
75. Desire to be healthier for my family

When You've Completed the Self-Evaluation . . .

Go back and look over your answers. Meet with a friend, spouse/partner, counselor, or with your accountability partner, and discuss the results. Ask yourself, "Why does this influence my motivation (for better or worse)?" Then, explain it out loud. Explaining it to someone else will help you better understand your exercise motivations. Use what you learn from this assessment to create your exercise for mental health goals and plan.

How Does Motivation Work:
Theory and Understanding

In order to understand our own motivations to implement and continue an exercise for mental health program, it's helpful to learn a little more about motivational theory and how motivation really works. There are numerous motivation theories (I recall taking a "Theories of Motivation" class in college that was three hours per week and lasted four months). This is not a book about motivation, and so we will not examine all the motivational theories. Instead, we will focus on three theories that, according to research, and in my opinion, are the most helpful when it comes to motivation in physical activity and exercise, especially exercise for mental health.

Self-Determination Theory

One of the most well-studied and validated motivational theories, when it comes to exercise, is called self-determination theory (SDT). Originally developed after years of research by Edward Deci and Richard Ryan, self-determination theory grew from a humanistic perspective, meaning that, similar to Abraham Maslow's Hierarchy of Needs (another, well-known theory of motivation) SDT focuses on the fulfillment of human needs, self-actualization, and how we can realize our potential as human beings (Teixeira et al., 2012). In short, self-determination theory posits that we are most motivated when our motivation comes from within—when we are self-motivated and self-determined.

Some of the key elements of self-determination include the following:

Intrinsic and Extrinsic Motivation
First, SDT differentiates between intrinsic and extrinsic motivation. Intrinsic motivation means doing something because we enjoy, are excited about, appreciate the challenge of, feel accomplished at, and/or like putting our skills to use in a given activity.

Examples of intrinsic motivation include someone who swims because she is talented and accomplished at it, someone who dances because he just loves to dance, or someone who enjoys the satisfaction she feels after rising to the challenge of a difficult workout. Each of these intrinsic motivators makes the activity itself worth doing, for different reasons but all of them internal and related directly to the activity.

On the flip side, extrinsic motivation refers to doing an activity to gain some form of outside reward. It involves a separate gain from that achieved by doing the activity for the activity's sake. For example, we may exercise to gain the approval or acceptance of others, earn a tangible reward like money or a treat when we're done, or because, if we don't participate, say, in a school physical education class, we'll get a bad grade. Extrinsic motivation can also involve our values and goals, such as someone who is motivated to exercise because he values becoming more muscular to feel better about his physical appearance (Ryan & Deci, 2000; Teixeira et al., 2012).

The best motivators for short-term activity are extrinsic motivators, but for long-term commitment, intrinsic motivation is key. Thus, we need to develop both if we want the optimal motivation to exercise for mental health.

Causality Orientations

Another element of self-determination theory, which goes along with internal and external motivation, is called "causality orientations"—a fancy term for the idea that we each have specific dispositional tendencies when it comes to motivation. These tendencies can impact our motivation to exercise, and keep at it.

Some of us are more internally oriented and more likely to follow our own thoughts, feelings, and courses of action. Others are more externally oriented, meaning they are more likely to follow external norms, advice, and directives. And some are generally "amotivated," meaning they're more likely to be unresponsive or passive to external or internal factors that might motivate their behavior (Teixeira et al., 2012). These differing orientations impact our beliefs, motivations, and practices of exercise for mental health (Markland, 2009). However, just because we have a tendency to act a certain way doesn't mean that we'll always act that way.

Understanding our "causal orientation" simply provides an invitation to be more self-aware about what might, or might not, drive and motivate us. Remember what we learned about practicing self-awareness? It can help us become more self-accepting, self-loving, and ultimately, can increase our sense of self-worth. We can then use this awareness to find ways to overcome or improve our motivational tendencies when they don't seem to be working well enough. (Review The Pyramid of Self-Worth from Key 2, for more on how practicing self-awareness can improve self-worth, and thus internal motivation.)

Basic Psychological Needs

The third element of self-determination theory that's useful when we're talking about exercise motivation is the human need for competence, relatedness, and autonomy (Ryan & Deci, 2000; Teixeira et al., 2012). We've already seen how feeling competent in activity is a huge predictor of sticking with an activity—for children, teens, and adults. Additionally, we've discussed how social interaction and connectedness are strong motivators for, as well as benefits of, exercise. When we talk about autonomy, we mean that people like doing what they like to do. When we enjoy the activity or feel some intrinsic reward for doing it, we're more likely to feel motivated to start and stick with it.

All three of these basic human needs combine to influence our exercise motivation, for better or worse. When we can identify our competence, relatedness, and autonomy needs concerning exercise for mental health, we can find ways to better meet those needs, thus improving our motivation.

Three Premises of Self-Determination Theory

Finally, self-determination theory is based on three premises, and these premises play an important role in exercise motivation. First is the premise that we humans are inherently proactive about seeking to master our internal world. This means we tend to work on developing and conquering our drives, thoughts, and emotions. This is a good thing when it comes to exercise for mental health, because if we want to master our internal world, then we're more likely to prioritize our mental health, and consequently, the strategies needed to "master" it, including exercise. Second, we tend toward growth, development, and integration. This means our natural tendency as humans is to want to improve and be whole. Third, however, is the premise that, though we may seek to master our internal world and inherently tend toward optimal actions and development, they don't happen automatically. We have to work at it (Ryan & Deci, 2000).

That's what this book is all about—working on new ways to master your internal world, or mental health, and seek the optional actions, like exercise, that will get you to your optimal development. The activity below, and others in this book, can show you how.

Self-Determination Theory and Exercise

Together, these qualities of self-determination theory, including our intrinsic and extrinsic motivators, causal orientation, our need for competence, enjoyment, and social interaction, and the three premises of SDT, can help us better understand exercise motivation and behavior. Studies show that intrinsic motivation is highly predictive of long-term exercise adherence, while extrinsic motivators, including how we look, fitness levels, and even health-related factors, are much less consistent (Teixeira et al., 2009). One study found that exercise motivation and adherence was significantly greater in those whose motives focused on competence, enjoyment, and social interaction than for those whose motives centered on appearance or fitness. Further, it showed that those who report that they enjoyed the exercise, post-workout, were far more likely to adhere to it than those who did not enjoy it (Ryan et al., 1997).

All of this provides an outline for how to increase exercise motivation. When we can increase enjoyment, competence, and social interaction, we will be more likely to exercise. When we seek to better understand our natural dispositional tendencies and find ways to strengthen intrinsic motivation, we're more likely to exercise. When we build on our innate tendency to want to grow and develop our internal world, then we will strengthen our motivation to exercise, and will thus be more likely to exercise—for mental health and for life.

Self-Determination Theory and You

What does all this mean for you? Understanding the principles of self-determination theory opens the door to greater self-understanding, and greater self-understanding opens the door to making change and increasing motivation. We'll discuss general strategies for increasing motivation, below, and strategies for overcoming specific roadblocks in Key 6, but right now, I want to encourage you to complete the following reflection questions on how these principles of self-determination theory impact you.

Reflection Questions:
Self-Determination Theory and You

1. What is your "causal orientation," or your natural dispositional tendency, when it comes to exercise? Are you more motivated by internal factors, like your own thoughts, beliefs, and feelings about exercise? Are you more motivated by external factors, like social interaction, accountability, and rewards? Or, are you more in the category of "amotivated"—more passive or unmoved by either internal or external rewards?

_____

_____

_____

_____

_____

_____

2. How does your orientation impact your desire, motivation, and actions to engage in physical activity?

_____

_____

_____

_____

_____

_____

3. How important are competence, enjoyment, and autonomy to you, in your life? How important are they in motivating you to exercise? Write about each of these.

_____

_____

_____

_____

_____

_____

_____

_____

4. What are your thoughts on the "three premises of self-determination theory," above? Do you believe you're "inherently proactive" when it comes to mastering your internal world—your mental health, emotions, drives, desires, feelings, thoughts, and behaviors? Why or why not?

_____

_____

_____

_____

_____

_____

_____

5. Do you feel naturally drawn toward growth and integration or is this more of a struggle for you? Why or why not?

_____

_____

_____

_____

_____

_____

6. Do you agree that these things don't just happen without
   hard work? Are you willing to do the work you need to
   do? Why or why not?

_____

_____

_____

_____

_____

_____

_____

_____

Expectancy Theory of Motivation

Expectancy theory looks at an essential component of motivation:
expectations. I've long quoted psychologist John Lund, who said,
"All frustration comes from unmet expectations" (2011). To his
wise words I add, "All frustration comes from *unrealistic* and *un-
communicated* (and therefore, unmet) expectations." Expectations
can make or break our choices—in relationships, self-worth,
achievement, and yes, exercise for mental health.

The expectancy theory of motivation, first proposed by Victor
Vroom, is based on the idea that people choose to act in a certain
way because of what they expect the result of their behavior to be. It
proposes that our motivation to behave is determined by the desir-
ability of the outcome that we expect that behavior to produce (Oliver, 1974). For example, if I expect that walking four days a week for

20 minutes will lead to less stress and greater happiness in my life, then I am much more likely to engage in that activity than I would be if, say, I expected that walking four days a week for 20 minutes would lead to me feeling even more exhausted than I already do.

Expectancy theory actually proposes a formula for motivation, based on three key elements: expectancy, instrumentality, and valence.

1. *Expectancy* refers to what we expect from our efforts. It says, "My effort will result in attaining my desired performance."
2. *Instrumentality* refers to the belief that our performance will lead to the desired outcome. It says, "I will receive my desired reward if I perform according to my expectations."
3. *Valence* looks at the value we place on the desired reward or outcome. It asks, "How much do I value that reward?"

The formula states that Motivation (M) is a product of Expectancy (E) times Instrumentality (I) times Valence (V), or M = E x I x V.

The Expectancy Theory and You

Though usually applied to work productivity and business situations, the expectancy theory formula has a valuable lesson for us, too—that if we want to feel motivated to exercise for mental health, then we have to evaluate our expectations. We need to understand what we believe will happen if we begin physical activity, to understand what our desired performance is, and whether or not this is realistic. Then, we need to know what rewards, or benefits, we're expecting and how valuable they are to us. When we can do these things, according to the expectancy theory formula, we can and will improve our motivation, and reduce our frustrations about exercise, as well. Remember: "All frustration comes from *unrealistic* and *un-communicated* expectations." Understanding our expectations is one way to communicate them to ourselves, and to make sure they're realistic.

Let's take a look at what the expectancy theory principles have to say about your expectations and motivations when it comes to exercise for mental health.

Ponder This . . . Expectancy Theory and You

Ask yourself:

1. What do I expect my performance to be when it comes to exercise?
2. What are the desired rewards that I expect from exercise?
3. How much do I value these desired rewards?
4. Overall, how realistic are my exercise expectations?

Four Simple Steps for Tackling Expectations

Many of us struggle to determine if our expectations are realistic or not. Clients often ask me to help them sort it out, saying, "I just can't tell what's realistic to expect." The following four steps can walk you through it:

1. *Identify your expectations.* Ask yourself, "What do I expect from this behavior, situation, or person?" Listen honestly, and give yourself plenty of time to hear and record the answers. If you feel stuck with this, then seek help from a trusted friend, family member, or counselor.
2. *Identify the current reality.* What's really going on with you right now? What are your current stressors, blocks, and challenges when it comes to exercise for mental health? What are your strengths? Take an honest look at your situation.
3. *Compare your expectations to your reality.* Ask yourself, "Is my expectation realistic in this situation?" Sometimes, the answer is "yes," but often the answer is "no." Does your reality match up with what you expect from exercise? For instance, do you expect an hour a day of uninterrupted, peaceful time to do yoga at home,

and yet the reality is you have young children and just feel frustrated because they keep interrupting? Or, do you expect to pick up running three miles a day and to feel energized by it, but the reality is you haven't exercised in years, your body can't handle the impact of running yet, and you end up quitting before you even get down the block?

4. *Either alter your expectation to match reality or alter reality to match your expectation.* For example, you might decide it's unrealistic to have calm yoga when you're home with your kids and opt for taking a class with childcare instead, or you might decide it's your expectations that are the problem and continue doing yoga at home, but when the kids come in, let them join you. Either way, you're bringing your expectations into line with your reality, and that boosts your motivation and effectiveness.

Identifying expectations gives us the opportunity to challenge, alter, and communicate them—to ourselves and to others—and that leads to a lot less frustration for everyone. Challenging and altering expectations boosts our motivation, and consequently helps us reach our exercise for mental health goals.

Do This . . . Tackle Expectations

Select one of the expectations you identified in "Ponder This," just above, and then, using the four steps for tackling expectations, try to understand if that expectation is realistic or not. Write about it in your journal, notebook, or digital device. Then, repeat for other expectations you discover.

Goal-Setting Theory of Motivation

Speaking of goals, now that we 1) understand the importance of intrinsic, or self-determined, motivation, and 2) know how to evaluate and alter our expectations, it's important to focus on goal-setting. Goal-setting is a fundamental part of motivation. Without some idea of the goal we're trying to achieve, who needs motivation in the first place? Goal-setting theory teaches us the principles that will help us set exercise for mental health goals that are motivating and effective.

Originally developed by Dr. Edwin Locke and later collaborated on by Dr. Gary Latham, goal-setting theory focuses on the important relationship between goals, motivation, and performance (Latham & Locke, 1991). Goal-setting theory asserts that motivation and performance will both be highest when individuals set goals that: 1) are specific, 2) difficult, but not too difficult, 3) help us evaluate our performance, and 4) are linked to feedback on how we did. These elements create greater commitment and acceptance in the goal-setter, and thus, greater motivation to complete the goal.

Studies show that 1) challenging goals are associated with a higher level of performance than easier goals; 2) specific goals lead to greater motivation and desired outcomes than telling yourself to just "do your best;" and 3) the choices we make are regulated by our intentions. In other words, we need to challenge ourselves to be specific, and to remember our intentions if we want to make choices that lead toward our goal of greater exercise participation. Additionally, studies show that deadlines and goals focused on learning something, rather than performance outcome, both increase goal-effectiveness. Group goal-setting can also be as effective as individual goal-setting (Locke, 1968; Locke et al., 1981; Lunenburg, 2011).

When we achieve something we've really had to work for, we feel a greater sense of accomplishment than we would have if we'd just done something easy. This is one reason why exercise can boost confidence and self-esteem—it can be challenging to get up and move every day, but when we do it, we feel good about ourselves. Tougher goals are actually more motivating, as long as they are not too tough, and as long as they are realistic. Sure, other things can motivate us, but Locke found that incentives like money, time limits, competition, and praise or criticism, were all mediated by the individual's goals and intentions. In other words, these incentives only work if they are in line with, or promote, our goals and intentions (Locke, 1968). It all goes back to goals, and Locke's now proven words: "an individual's conscious ideas regulate his actions" (Locke et al., 1981).

If we're seeking to take action with exercise, then it would be vital to know what our "conscious ideas" about exercise are, right? To be clear on our intentions, and to create specific goals that outline what we're hoping to accomplish? According to goal-setting theory, this is exactly what we need in order to be effectively motivated when it comes to any activity, and that includes physical activity.

Reflection Questions: Goal-setting

1. Have you set goals for your mental health? If so, are they specific and challenging, but not too difficult? Do they motivate you toward greater mental health? If not, what has prevented you so far?

_____

_____

_____

_____

_____

2. Have you outlined goals for regular physical activity or exercise? If so, are they specific and challenging? Do you feel motivated by your goals? If not, what has prevented you from setting goals so far?

_____

_____

_____

_____

_____

Goal-Setting Strategies

There are five basic principles in goal-setting theory: clarity, challenge, commitment, feedback, and task complexity (Pavey, 2015). Using these principles, we can set exercise goals that are achievable and boost our motivation. Let's look more in depth at each principle and see how we can apply it to exercise for mental health goal-setting.

1. **Clarity.** Our goals need to be clear, understandable, and preferably written down. In order to be clear with our exercise goals, we need to give ourselves time to ponder our needs, desires, and what we're hoping to gain from exercise. Use the tools above, from self-determination theory and expectancy theory, to get clear on where you currently are and where you desire to be. Then, set specific goals that will help you get there.

   Example: Instead of writing, "I want to exercise more," write, "I will swim for 20 minutes, two mornings a week, and walk with my family after work for 20 minutes, three days a week." The clearer we can make our goals, the more we will know how to achieve them.

2. **Challenge.** Again, we need goals that push us. Nothing too difficult or unattainable, but set goals that challenge *you*. Remember, what is challenging to you might not be challenging to someone else, and vice versa. That's okay. The main goal is to be honest, to compare ourselves only to ourselves and never to other people when it comes to exercise for mental health.

   Example: If you're very new to exercise, then you might start with a goal to simply walk around the block three days a week. That might not seem like a challenge for some, but for others, it's a huge step—literally. Later, you might challenge yourself by setting the goal to walk around the neighborhood, and eventually the challenge might be walking a mile or two, five days a week. The point is to do what will challenge you, while also making it attainable.

3. **Commitment.** When setting goals, we need to spell out what our commitment will be. Write down how often you will exercise,

what you will do, how long each session will be, who will exercise with you, and give yourself a time period for when you will evaluate your goals.

Example: "I'll go to the climbing gym with my friend every Saturday morning for an hour, and I'll play basketball with my family twice a week, for at least 30 minutes. I will do these things for one month and then check in to see if I need to reevaluate my goals." It doesn't matter if you commit to a week, or a month, or six months—what matters is that you commit, and that you put your commitment in writing.

4. **Feedback.** We need to check in with ourselves regularly, to revisit our goals and make sure they're still in line with our intentions. Additionally, we feel most motivated when we receive feedback from others. Ask your spouse or your best friend to read over your goals and to be a support for you. Check in with them and listen to what they have to say. If you go to a gym or work with a fitness professional, his or her feedback can be helpful, too. No matter what, make sure you provide a way to give yourself feedback when you're setting goals.

   Example: "I will review my goals every Sunday and ask myself, 'How am I doing with this goal? How is this goal working for me? Do I need to revise my goals? Or, am I feeling good about where I am?'" Then, follow through with your feedback plan. You can also do this with an exercise partner, or ask your trainer or a friend to give feedback on your progress and motivation, once a week, for example.

5. **Task complexity.** Regularly check in on the complexity of the tasks you've set up in your goals, to make sure they don't become too complex or overwhelming.

   Example: If you've set a goal to rollerblade with friends twice a week and do a high-intensity fitness class three times a week and you pull a muscle in your leg, you're going to have to re-evaluate. Circumstances change, and we need to be flexible. The important thing is to stick with the goals, even when we need to change them. For instance, while your leg is healing, perhaps you could try swimming, rowing, lifting weights, or playing catch with your kids.

SMART Goal-Setting

Another tool for goal-setting is the commonly known mnemonic, SMART, which stands for: Specific, Measurable, Attainable, Results-Focused, and Time-bound. Let's use SMART and the five principles above to help you create effective, motivating exercise for mental health goals. As we outline each component of SMART, use the lines provided to answer the questions given. At the end, you will have a pretty thorough set of goals to get you started on your exercise for mental health plan.

1. **Specific:** As we saw in the research above, specific, clearly outlined goals are central to staying motivated and achieving those goals. To make goals specific, I suggest using the question words, "Who, What, Why, Where, When, and How?"

   Who? "Who will be involved in my exercise goals? Will I involve my family, friends, a workout buddy, an online support group, or do I prefer to exercise on my own? Will I incorporate others into my feedback plan? If so, whom?"

   _____

   _____

   _____

   _____

   _____

   Remember that whether you exercise in a group, with a partner, or on your own, it's still helpful to have someone to whom you are accountable, who will "check in" with you and cheer you on. So, ask yourself, "Who will be my accountability and/or feedback partner(s)?"

   _____

   _____

   _____

   _____

What? "What types of exercise will I do? What motivational strategies might I employ to help me, based on the ideas presented above?" This could include taking a class, family activities, increasing steps taken each day, or stretching each night. The possibilities are endless when it comes to physical activity, so be sure to select activities you're likely to enjoy and do.

_____

_____

_____

_____

_____

_____

Where? "Where do I plan to exercise? At home? At a gym? In my community? Outside? Inside?"

_____

_____

_____

When? "When will I exercise?" List the days of the week you intend to exercise, how often you plan to exercise, for how long, and give a time commitment for your exercise goals.

_____

_____

_____

_____

_____

Why? "What are my specific reasons, my purpose, or the benefits of setting and accomplishing this goal to exercise?" Remind yourself of the long-term vision you have for your health and mental-emotional-social-spiritual well-being. Go back and revisit the list of physical and mental health benefits in Key 1 and the list of self-worth and family benefits from keys 2 and 3 and include those that stand out most to you. Also include those values that impact your desire to exercise, dreams, hopes, and anything that influences why you are setting these goals.

_____

_____

_____

_____

_____

_____

_____

_____

_____

_____

2. **Measurable:** Set goals that you can measure. This goes along with the "clarity" principle, above. Look at the items you wrote down in step one. How can you form these into measurable goals? This might include things like, "I will keep a weekly calendar and write down how long I exercise each day," or "I will use a pedometer to track my steps each day," or "I will use a fitness app to track my progress."

_____

_____

_____

_____

_____

_____

_____

3. **Attainable:** Again, be realistic. Revisit the suggestions for realistic expectations, and the concept of "task complexity," above, and then use those principles to make sure you are setting realistic goals. It's okay to recognize our own weaknesses and needs and say, "This is too much, at least for now." Eventually, you can work up to the toughest goals you have in mind, but for now,

remember: challenging but not too challenging. Write about whether your goals are attainable or not. If they're not, how will you change them?

_____

_____

_____

_____

_____

_____

4. **Relevant:** Goals should be relevant to the direction you want your life to ultimately take. When it comes to exercise for mental health, it's important to remember your ultimate desired outcomes: greater mental health, happiness, confidence, and so forth. Keeping these things in mind will keep your goals streamlined with what you most desire to achieve. Ask yourself, "Are the goals I'm working on now in line with what I hope for my future? Will they get me where I want to be? If so, how? If not, why not and what can I do to improve them?"

_____

_____

_____

_____

_____

_____

5. **Time-Bound:** Give yourself a deadline for every goal you set. As the research states, deadlines help us feel more motivated. Just make sure your deadline is realistic. With exercise for mental health, you'll probably want to set deadlines of a few weeks or months at a time, and then to check in and set new goals to keep you exercising for life. Ask yourself, "What is my deadline for the goals I'm setting today? Is it a realistic timeline for me to achieve? Why or why not?"

_____

_____

_____

_____

_____

_____

_____

_____

_____

These goal-setting strategies can be used for setting mental health goals, too. For example, if you want to feel less depressed and are in a place where you are able to motivate yourself, you might set a SMART goal of "I will go for a walk for 10 minutes every morning, because I know it will lift my mood. I will keep track by making a note on my smartphone calendar when I've completed it and check in with myself every day after I get back to see how I'm feeling and if my mood has improved. I will do this for one month and check in each week with myself, and my wife, to see how I'm progressing in reaching this goal."

Yes, it's a long goal. But yes, it incorporates all the elements of goal-setting, and it's much more likely to be accomplished when it is SMART.

Reflection Questions: Mental Health Goals

What are your mental health goals? Are you seeking to overcome something like anxiety, stress, or grief? Are you focused on becoming your true, best self, by developing greater self-worth? Are you seeking flourishing through greater joy, peace, love, and meaning in everyday life? Or, all three? Take a few minutes to ponder what you're seeking when it comes to mental health, and then write down your thoughts on the lines provided below. Using these reflections, go back and apply the SMART and other goal-setting principles, above, to help you write down your mental health goals.

_____
_____
_____
_____
_____
_____
_____
_____
_____
_____
_____
_____

Get Motivated, Feel Confident: Tyler's Story

Tyler is a 38-year-old, married father of three who grew up in an active family. He ran long-distance track and swam in high school, and has enjoyed many outdoor physical activities throughout his life.

As he became a father, and as his family and work responsibilities grew, however, Tyler found it harder and harder to exercise, and for a long time he did no physical activity. He realized he needed start exercising again, and he knew that, for him, that meant going to the gym. But, he felt so embarrassed about his body that he told himself he first needed to workout at home, so he could lose some weight, before he could dare show up at the gym. For Tyler, the struggle to go to the gym was real. He had to want it before he could make himself go; no one else could want it for him. When to go, making time to go, being excited to go has been a continual process.

But he was eventually able to make himself go. How?

First, Tyler joined an online fitness training program, which made him accountable, a huge plus for Tyler. This motivated him, but he still compared himself to the other participants and felt discouraged he wasn't making the same progress as quickly as they were. This translated to self-doubt that made it even tougher to get out of bed in the morning to exercise, far earlier than he needed to just to get to work every day. The time commitment was extremely tough, especially when time was so scarce between work, family, church, and other commitments.

Second, Tyler started scheduling exercise. He realized that morning was not the best time for him to exercise and switched to stopping by the gym after work. This helped him decompress and de-stress from the day before coming home to his family.

Third, Tyler set achievable goals. Since he's a "make-a-list" guy, Tyler started writing down specific, achievable goals for when he would work out and what exactly he would do. For instance, "Do x workout, with x reps, with x weight." When he began, his goals focused on weight loss, but as he's changed and adjusted these goals, they now focus on "lifestyle improvements," including eating nutritious foods, with specific goals. "I started with, 'Don't eat candy after workouts,' and then progressed to, 'Eat three vegetables a day,' and now, "Eat foods that build muscle and make me feel good."

Fourth, Tyler learned to "mix it up." He keeps focused and motivated by mixing things up with different types of exercises on different days. "I've 'graduated' from exercising at home to working out at the gym," he says. "But it is not a social event. I'm there to work, and I try to keep myself motivated." Some days, he opts for a run instead of hitting the gym. Some days, it still feels like a challenge to do anything, but now that he knows the payoffs of exercise—on his confidence, body, and mind—he looks for new ways to keep exercise fresh and motivating.

Fifth, Tyler focused on being positive. "Attitude is key," he says. He wasn't always happy when exercising, and he has had to work very hard for many years to get to the place where he says he now enjoys exercise. He credits this enjoyment to developing a good attitude about exercise. He now knows he feels physically and mentally better when he exercises. "I may struggle physically with the exercises, but I feel good when I'm done. I felt the emotional results before I saw the physical results."

Finally, Tyler has become a partner in exercise with his wife. Though he used to feel insecure exercising with her, because she seemed more naturally suited to exercise, Tyler now considers her his biggest asset. "We don't always exercise together or eat the same foods, but we hold each other accountable. We set each other up for success, and she encourages, lifts, and pushes (sometimes pulls) me to achieve my goals. We make a great team."

A Few Final Goal-Setting Tips

The more I work with clients like Tyler, and the more I talk with friends, the more I keep seeing the same pattern emerge—that at our core, male or female, we all just want to feel confident, belong, and reach our potential. Setting clear goals can lead us to our potential. They can help us apply and achieve all the things we're discussing here in this book. The right goals can form us into who we desire to be.

Here are a few more suggestions to make goal-setting as effective as possible for you.

Create a Vision of Success

Stephen Covey, author of the bestseller, *The Seven Habits of Highly Effective People,* said it best: "Begin with the end in mind" (2013). Too often, we set a goal without a clear vision of what a "successful" outcome might look like. We know we want greater mental health, for instance, but what, exactly, does that entail? Before you set a goal, get clear on the best end result. Close your eyes and envision how you would like to think, feel, behave, or be after your goal is achieved. Write it down. Then, write down what success for each goal would look like to you. (We'll discuss how to create an "exercise for mental health vision" in Key 8.)

Don't Try to Do Too Much at Once

It may seem impressive to set 10 exercise or mental health goals, but you can't really work on them all at once. You're better off to try one or two at a time, and add more as you feel ready.

Don't Expect Change to Come Too Quickly

Often, we set a goal and say, "I'm starting tomorrow," and then dive in. While that can sometimes work, more often we're frustrated because we find ourselves slipping by day three. Instead, we need to realize that change is a process that can take longer than we'd like. There's much more to making lasting change than we think, as you'll see in Key 5. So, give yourself time.

Don't Quit if You "Fail"

I put "fail" in quotes, because frequently, what we think of as failure really isn't. The only true failure is quitting. Lasting change and growth usually takes several tries, and readjusting our goals as we make mistakes is part of a successful outcome. We'll discuss this more in Key 5, but in the meantime, don't quit on your goals. Readjust. Reevaluate. Rewrite, but don't quit.

Take the Time to Create a Solid Plan

Don't jump in to the "action" phase of a goal before you've taken the time to contemplate and prepare properly. As we will discuss in the next key, there are actually six stages of change, and skipping steps won't help you get where you want to be any sooner. Instead, think about your vision and the steps it will take to get there. What challenges do you anticipate and how might you overcome them? What time frame is best for this goal, and how will you know when you've achieved it? Write all of this down, creating a plan you can follow to achieve your goal.

Write Goals in the Positive
and Use the Active Present Tense

Instead of telling yourself what not to do, tell yourself what to do. Instead of saying, "I will not be lazy," say, "I am increasing physical activity everyday." It helps you feel more empowered and focused on how to achieve your goal. And, speaking in the present helps your mind act as if you have already achieved your goal. It helps you believe in yourself, reminding you of what you are capable.

Make Yourself Accountable and Stick With It

If we have no accountability, it's going to be hard to stay the course when things get tough. Some of us are great with holding ourselves accountable–checking in, reevaluating, encouraging, and sticking with it on your own–but many are not. According to research, most people do best by having a partner to help achieve goals. Consider setting up a buddy system with a friend or family member, like Tyler has done with his wife, where you check in and encourage each other regularly. Involve your partner or even the whole family by helping everyone set one or two goals and then working to achieve them together. Post a goal on Facebook and encourage friends to ask about it. Or, join my Exercise 4 Mental Health Facebook group (exercise4mentalhealth.com) for a built-in support system. However you do it, if you make yourself accountable–to yourself and to someone else–you're more likely to stick with and eventually achieve your goals.

Healthy Self-Evaluation

One more important tool to increase motivation is healthy self-evaluation. I say, "healthy," because when it comes to exercise and mental health, our self-evaluations can be anything but healthy.

Self-evaluation shouldn't involve pointing out every "bad" thing we think, feel, or do. It isn't about beating ourselves up when we don't do things right—when we're not motivated, succumb to fatigue, laziness, or fear, or don't exercise like we know we should. Self-doubt, self-criticism, and self-contempt only lead to self-defeat. These are not part of healthy self-evaluation.

Healthy self-evaluation is taking an honest, loving look at how we're doing. It's about seeing the reality so we can gauge our progress and make change as needed and desired. When it comes to exercise for mental health, healthy self-evaluation is an especially critical skill to develop, because it allows us to: 1) evaluate our progress in the most beneficial, healthy ways; 2) pay attention to what is and is not motivating us, as well as to roadblocks that stand in our way; and 3) overcome the negative, self-defeating thoughts and feelings that drag us down and lead to giving up.

How do we develop "healthy self-evaluation?" Tools like those we've learned in The Pyramid of Self-Worth help us understand our true nature and learn to see all sides of who we are. As we practice these skills, we develop greater self-worth, and this helps us be gentle and fair with ourselves when it comes to self-evaluation. Also, the ideas we've just discussed, on self-determination, expectancy, and goal-setting theories of motivation, can help us develop healthy self-evaluation. As we practice identifying our intrinsic and extrinsic motivators, challenging and changing expectations, and setting realistic, achievable goals, we will strengthen a realistic, well balanced, and hopeful view of ourselves.

Additionally, when it comes to healthy self-evaluation, we need to understand how to check in with ourselves regularly, to self-monitor without self-criticizing. Key 5 is all about how to identify, challenge, and change faulty thoughts, beliefs, and self-talk, but the following strategies will also help—if we practice diligently.

1. *Develop a habit of checking in with yourself regularly.* Again, your focus is self-evaluation—seeing all sides of your exercise and mental health

2. *Schedule a weekly check in time.* This is a time to monitor your progress for the week, to see what worked and what didn't work to

keep your motivated to exercise, and to reevaluate your goals as needed. You might want to use a journal to keep track of your weekly progress and write about your experiences. I find that journaling helps me cut to the core of the issues, better understand blocks and problems, and just vent things out when I'm feeling frustrated or overwhelmed.

3. *Practice self-monitoring before and after exercise.* Check in with how you're feeling, then take a brief walk around the block. Check back in and see how you feel. Do you feel better? Worse? The same? Why or why not? Practice doing this often, and once you find the exercise program that is right for you, this skill will be valuable in reminding you of the benefits you'll receive, even when you don't feel motivated to exercise. It can be a great way to get yourself up and moving anyway.

4. *Learn how to recognize the mental health benefits of exercise.* First, learn about the mental health benefits (see Key 1), and then, use self-monitoring to see how they apply to you.

Get Motivated

I realize there are a lot of different theories, suggestions, and strategies in this key. They are here to help you, and it's important that you use them in the ways that feel most useful. I hope you'll at least answer the questions and do the activities I've offered in this key, because I really do believe they can make a difference. Give each principle a try. But beyond that, it's up to you how you apply these things to increase the motivation in your life—motivation to exercise, improve your mental health, and achieve the long-term vision and goals you desire.

Next, we delve into your thoughts and beliefs—they are critical when it comes to exercise for mental health motivation and success.

CHANGE HOW YOU THINK ABOUT EXERCISE

"Don't limit yourself. Many people limit themselves to what they think they can do. You can go as far as your mind lets you. What you believe, remember, you can achieve."

—Mary Kay Ash

I know you're probably dying to get started on an exercise plan, but it's not time just yet. As you will learn in this key, we must first prepare before we can take action, and mental preparation is essential.

In Key 4, I promised that we would work on changing your thoughts and beliefs, and that's exactly what this key is all about. It's about preparing your mind for exercise. It's about building the mental skills and tools you need to feel motivated, overcome roadblocks, and stay dedicated to exercise for life. It's about getting off our "buts"—our, "But I don't have time to exercise," "But I'm too tired," or "But my body's just not made for exercise." No more "buts." This key is about deciding to make positive change, and to leave all the "buts" behind.

One way to think of it is like trying to re-route a river with boulders in its way. You can't change the river's flow unless you first change the underlying structure of the riverbed (Fritz, 1989). That's exactly what we're seeking to do in this key—to change the fundamental structure of your thoughts, feelings, and beliefs about exercise for mental health so they can better support the flow of healthy exercise behavior in your life.

First, we'll learn a new way to view exercise "failure" and "success." Then, we'll learn how to challenge and change faulty thoughts and beliefs. These skills can help you overcome roadblocks, set goals that work, and keep you exercising for life. Additionally, these tools are some of the most effective for treating depression, anxiety, and a number of other mental health issues. You'll benefit not only by becoming dedicated to exercise, but also by applying these skills to other areas of your life to help you overcome, become, and flourish.

Change Your Beliefs
About Exercise = Change Your Life

It is possible to change thoughts and beliefs that feed negative emotions and block exercise success. I know, because I've not only done it in my own life; I've helped individuals, couples, and families learn to do so, too.

One couple, Tammy and Matt, came to me in the midst of a major crisis. Tammy, for reasons she couldn't explain, had suddenly quit her bipolar disorder medication, cold turkey—a common occurrence in people with severe psychiatric illness. This created an intense and pervasive earthquake in Tammy and Matt's lives as Tammy experienced significant mania, with symptoms of lying and deceiving that were completely uncharacteristic. Matt stood by her through these painful days, even as she tried to push him away with her lies, and he remained through the dark days of depression that followed. This went on for over a year, and it took a severe toll on both individuals, their relationship, and their three children.

When Tammy and Matt found me, Tammy had slowly been stabilized, back on the medication, and they had seen several different doctors and therapists, but none of the approaches had worked. They were on the brink of divorce. Tammy was beating herself up because she had caused so much distress to her husband and children, and Matt was harboring resentment from all he had endured during her manic-depressive episodes. The biggest blocks were that Tammy wasn't yet able to identify her self-defeating thoughts, and Matt wasn't yet able to identify his resentments. Both were suffering from negative thinking and feelings that were controlling their minds, emotions, and marriage, and they couldn't seem to understand, stop, and alter the very thoughts and beliefs that were steering them toward disaster.

Have you ever felt down on yourself because of how you feel, think, or behave? Have you ever had trouble forgiving others for the pain they've brought into your life? Have you ever felt like your feelings are standing in the way of what you want most—like greater mental health, stronger relationships, and a happy family? Can you relate to the idea of unidentified thoughts or negative self-talk that wreaks havoc on your feelings, behavior, and/or life? Have you ever found it difficult to change?

I would wager almost all of us have experienced these things, and in some way or another, we can all relate to Tammy and Matt. We'll hear more about them later, but first, let's learn a few important things about making lasting change.

Six Steps to Lasting Change

How do we make lasting change? That's the big question, because change is hard. We make it even harder on ourselves when we don't understand the nature of change and don't have the necessary skills to identify, challenge, and change the things we need to in our lives.

Below, I've outlined six steps to lasting change, including a new way to understand change and some of the most effective tools for implementing change, based on CBT. Work through these steps slowly, making sure you take in each principle and apply it in the activities provided. Give yourself the gift of lasting change by learning the steps it takes to get there.

Step 1: Understand the Spiral of Change

One of the most frequent questions I hear as a psychologist is, "Why is it so hard to change?" Most of us want to change the bad habits, negative emotions, depressing circumstances, and weaknesses we've been given. Most of us believe that changing these things is possible. Most of us, I daresay, even believe it's possible to overcome the roadblocks to exercise success. However, do we believe we not only can, but also that we *will* do these things? Do we believe we have what it takes to make lasting positive change?

Change is a fundamental part of life. If you need proof, just look at your body. Do you still look, feel, or act like you did when you were an infant? Of course not (or, hopefully, not the "act" part anyway). Our bodies change, circumstances, and minds change, but are *we* choosing to change and progress? Are we seeking personal growth, or simply waiting for change to happen to us? When we're talking about changing the way we think and feel about exercise for mental and physical health, we must be willing to choose to act—now.

Change is hard for different reasons. Sometimes we're not fully convinced that change is needed. Sometimes we know we need to change but aren't sure how. Sometimes we're trying to change and think we know how, but it's just not sticking. I see this all the time in my psychology practice—a desire for change, but a lack of understanding and skills to make that change work.

The Transtheoretical Model of Change

One of the most helpful concepts I've found to explain the process of change is The Transtheoretical Model of Change, by James Prochaska, Ph.D. (Prochaska, Norcross, & DiClemente, 2007). Most of us think that change is about deciding to do something differently, and then doing it. But what Prochaska teaches is that there are actually six stages involved in changing and forming healthier habits. He shows us that change, in fact, works more like a spiral staircase than an escalator, and that we may go up and down that spiral several times before we make it to the top.

First, let's explore the six stages of change. Then we'll see what we can learn from them.

> *Stage 1: Precontemplation.* *"I don't yet recognize I have a need for change; others may see it, but I don't."* Friends and family may be telling you that you need to exercise. They may say, "It will help your mental health and make you feel better about yourself." It might have even briefly crossed your mind, too, but you're not convinced. I like to say that, right now, we're all in the precontemplation stage for something!
>
> *Stage 2: Contemplation.* *"I know I need to change, but . . . ."* In stage two, we realize the need for change and start thinking about it. We may talk to our family and friends about our need for exercise, but we're not yet ready to make a plan or to take action.
>
> *Stage 3: Preparation.* *"I will implement my plan for change within the next month."* In stage three, we know we need to change and we're preparing to take action. This may involve doing research, such as looking into the mental health benefits of different physical activities, strengthening our motivations for exercise, and setting specific, realistic goals. In this stage, we intend to take action and implement our plan within the next few weeks or month.
>
> *Stage 4: Action.* *"I am actively working on making change."* Stage four is when we finally get to work. This includes implementing the plan we've made and evaluating our progress as we go. Stage four is the long, hard part of making change. It's where we finally put our thoughts and plans into place and see what happens. Sometimes we find that our original plan works, and change starts to happen. Other times we realize we need to go back to the drawing board and create a new, more effective plan.
>
> *Stage 5: Maintenance.* *"I've achieved the change I wanted, but now I need to make sure it lasts."* In order for change to persist, we need a plan to maintain what we've gained. In the case of exercise, we need a lifelong strategy to keep us moving and

reaping the benefits. We need to be willing to work through the roadblocks that come our way, like boredom, and find innovative ways to keep our momentum going, like trying new physical activities to keep things fresh.

Stage 6: Termination. "I am permanently changed. I no longer need a maintenance plan." Truth is, most of us will never reach this stage for many of the changes we make, and that's okay. It's part of the nature of change to keep working on it. Sure, it's possible to completely quit a bad habit and never need to work on it again, like when you were a kid and finally stopped biting your nails. But, the majority of changes will never reach termination. Even if change really is permanent, most of the time, it's because we're maintaining it well.

Five Lessons from the Transtheoretical Model of Change

What can we learn from the Transtheoretical Model of Change to help us create a habit of exercise for mental health?

1. *Simply deciding to change, and actually changing, is rare.* You can't expect to change at the snap of your fingers. Though it's certainly been known to happen for some, it's not likely for most. Have patience with yourself as you work on making exercise part of your life. When you make mistakes, give yourself a break. Then, get up and try again.

2. *Trying to accomplish changes you're not ready for sets you up for failure.* One of the biggest mistakes people make when trying to change is failing to admit they're not ready. Change requires giving something up in order to gain something new and, hopefully, better. All change requires a loss, however. Even if we know we need to start walking three times a week, for example, it can be tough to let go of our habit of not walking, if for no other reason than our habits are comfortable, we're used to them, and they're easy. It's one thing to know you need to change; it's another to be ready to let yourself change. The spiral of change shows us there are three steps before we take action, and two more after.

3. *If you want successful change, you need to know which stage you're*

in. Too many of us jump into the "action" stage before we're ready. Taking the time to first analyze which stage of change you're in can dramatically improve your success.

4. *The Six Stages of Change work like a spiral staircase, and most people spiral several times.* Most self-changers cycle up and down the spiral several times before change sticks. Moving up, down, and back up in the spiral of change is all part of the process.

5. *As long as you are in the spiral, you are progressing—it doesn't matter which way you are headed!* Research shows that people who take action but "fail" within the next month are twice as likely to succeed over the next six months than those who don't take action at all (Prochaska, Norcross, & Declemente, 2007). Prochaska calls this "recycling." For example, keeping your goal of jogging every day, for seven days straight, and then failing to jog for the next two weeks, may feel like failure. But as long as you recycle to the preparation stage—as long as you create a new plan of action—you're still succeeding. Without the "failure" of the jogging plan, you might never have taken action on a new "go for a walk with a friend" plan that eventually moves you to "maintenance." Success is staying in and working in the spiral of change, no matter where you are in the spiral or which way you're currently moving.

The Transtheoretical Model of Change helps me understand that change really is more complex than I once believed. It helps me understand what to focus on in order to change my habits and myself. It helps me let go of the frustration I feel when change isn't happening quickly enough, and helps me see that maybe what I once saw as "failure" was really just a step on my way to the top of the spiral. I believe it can do the same for you—if you allow it to.

Reflection Questions: Spiral of Change

1. When it comes to making exercise a regular part of your life, which stage of change do you believe you are in—

precontemplation, contemplation, preparation, action, maintenance, or termination?

_____
_____
_____
_____
_____
_____

2. What is one thing you can do to begin to move from your current stage to the next stage of change? How might you take that step?

_____
_____
_____
_____
_____
_____

3. How do you define "failure" in your pursuit of exercise for mental health? How do you define "success"?

_____
_____
_____
_____
_____
_____

4. Can you expand your views of failure and success to include the principles from the spiral of change? If so, which concepts are most helpful to you?

_____
_____
_____
_____

_____

_____

Step 2: Learn the Thought Cycle

One of the most validated psychotherapy methods for changing your mind, mood, and mental health is CBT. Cognitive-behavioral therapy is a structured, short-term method that focuses on solving problems and changing unhealthy, or unhelpful, thoughts and behaviors. I mentioned it several times in Key 1, since it's considered one of the most effective treatments for many mental health disorders.

The premise of CBT is that our thoughts, feelings, bodily responses, and behaviors are all connected and influence one another. It works like a cycle: we have a thought, the thought creates an emotion (or two, or three), our emotions cause our body to respond (i.e. heart rate increases, we get flushed), and all of these contribute to our behavior. Then, our behavior influences our next thoughts, and the cycle continues. Here's a simple diagram explaining how this works:

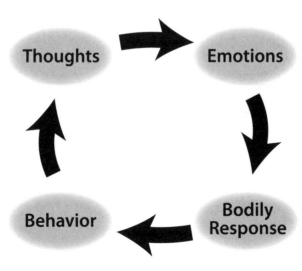

Fig. 2 Thought Cycle Example

The majority of our thoughts are what we call "automatic thoughts," meaning they happen automatically. We don't ponder or even hear them most of the time; they come without warning, and often without intention. Yet, these thoughts still set off the same cycle, influencing our emotions, body, and behavior. Just think of what these automatic thoughts could do to you if they remained unheard and unchecked.

Let's say you just woke up, it's your day off, and you're trying to decide what to do today. Your thoughts may sound like, "I should get up and go for a walk. It's supposed to be a beautiful day, and exercise is good for my body and mood." You feel calm and hopeful, your body is relaxed, you are breathing nice and steady, and you slowly roll over to get out of bed. However, it's so cozy in your bed that your thoughts shift: "But, I'm so comfy here in my soft bed, and I really could use some extra sleep." You might notice additional thoughts like, "I really do need to sleep more, because I've been so stressed about work and lately. Now that I think about it, I have so much to do today I don't have time for exercise or sleep. Ugh! I feel like I can't breathe, I'm so stressed about my life!" Your emotions may start off relaxed and sleepy, and then move to feeling guilty for not exercising, and then anxious about your to-do list. Your body responds by getting tense — heart rate increasing, breathing becoming shallow. And your behavior? You angrily jump out of bed and head to the kitchen, where you open a box of donuts and try to eat your way out of your stress.

Sound familiar? Even if you haven't been in this exact situation, it's easy to see how our thoughts can create, or add to, stress, bad moods, and more problems overall than we ever intended. Not only did the person in this example not exercise, he didn't sleep in, and he ended up starting the day with stress and donuts. The worst part is, unless we stop and intervene, the cycle will continue. His next thoughts will likely be, "I can't believe I just ate that whole box of donuts! I can't even take care of my body, so how am I supposed to take care of my home, work, and family?" What started off as a pleasant, positive wake up, with intentions to exercise and enjoy the day, ended in a sugar crash that also crashed his mood and self-esteem.

Of course, it's hard to hear, challenge, and change unwanted or unhealthy thoughts. Like any new skill it takes practice, so it's best to start with small, realistic steps. First, take the time to digest how this thought cycle works. Then, you can learn how to make it work for you.

Ponder This . . .

How have you experienced the thought cycle in your own life? Can you relate to the example above or to something similar? Think of an example of when your thoughts might have affected your feelings, body, and behavior, and keep it in mind as we work through the remaining steps.

Step 3: Use a Thought Record to Identify Thoughts and Emotions

One of my favorite tools for changing thoughts and beliefs is called a thought record. The thought record is a CBT tool that can help you break into a thought cycle. It's purpose is to help you discover underlying thoughts and beliefs that create emotional distress, challenge those thoughts and beliefs, and then change them, thus changing your feelings, body, and behavior. When used correctly, the principles learned from a thought record can literally change your life.

How to Use a Thought Record

Below is an example of a thought record. You may use the one in this book, photocopy it for your use, or download one from http://www.exercise4mentalhealth.com. You'll notice there are seven columns. For now, we'll only be using the first five.

Thought Record, Part 1

Date	Situation Briefly Describe: *"What's going on?"*	Automatic Thought(s) *"What do I hear myself saying?"* *"What's going through my head?"* *"What sentences do I hear?"* Write your stream of automatic thoughts.	Emotion(s) *"What am I feeling?"* Identify/list emotions— sad, angry, frustrated . . . (There are usually more than one.)	Rate Rate the emotion, from 1-10. *"How powerful are my feelings?"*

Christina G. Hibbert, Psy.D. 2013
www.DrChristinaHibbert.com

Use this thought record whenever you're faced with powerful situations and emotions, like when you're feeling stressed, overwhelmed, depressed, or anxious. You can even use the thought record when you're feeling especially joyful or "up" and want to better understand what helped you feel this way. As you listen, you'll begin to hear patterns of thought that feed into how you feel and what you do. You'll begin to notice the impact your thoughts have on your life. You'll write them all down, challenge them, and then you'll have the power to change them.

For the purposes of this book, I would like you to pay particular attention to those situations and emotions related to exercise, your body, and your mental health. However, a thought record can help you in any area of your life—with overcoming mental illness, stress, and life challenges, with becoming who you desire to be, and with flourishing—so use it as often as you wish. Here's how to start:

1. *Date—Write down the date of each significant experience.* At first, it's common to write things down well after the situation is over—later that day, the next day, a couple days after—so just do your best to remember the correct date. Eventually, you'll be writing things down in the middle of the situation, or even before.

2. *Situation—Briefly describe what was happening at the time.* It can be as simple as, "I was telling my co-worker I was going to start jogging after work and he laughed at me. " Or, "I got on the treadmill and felt like I just couldn't do it."

3. *Automatic thoughts—Listen to your thoughts and write them down.* First, try to hear the thousands of thoughts that float through your mind. Throughout the day, stop and listen. It's important to hear what you're saying to yourself to ensure you're able to capture it all on your thought record. Your thoughts will sound like sentences: "I should go to the gym." "I'm too tired and stressed." "I can't make myself do anything. I'm such a loser!" It may sound harsh, but you'd be surprised what kinds of thoughts we allow in our minds—at least, until we hear them. Write them all down. Then, you can work to change them.

4. *Emotion—Pay attention to what you're feeling and write it all down.*

After you've learned to hear your thoughts, it's time to focus on your emotions. Emotions are usually one or two words, and there's a much smaller list of possible emotions than thoughts. When identifying emotions, it helps to ask, "What do I feel right now?" Then, list as many emotions as you can discern. Sad, happy, angry, frustrated, calm, at peace, anxious, stressed, worried, afraid, content, loved, healthy—the list of possible emotions goes on, and usually, you'll be feeling more than one in any given situation. Identify as many emotions as you can. One thing that can make this tough, especially at first, is that thoughts and emotions are often highly intertwined and can become so fused together, they feel like a jumbled mess. It can be difficult to tease apart the thoughts from the underlying emotions. Just work on hearing the sentences (thoughts) in your head and then paying attention to your body to learn how you feel (emotions). As you practice, you'll get a feel for the difference between thoughts and emotions, and you will see how much easier it is to understand each when they're teased apart. A video demonstration from my website, http://www.exercise4mental health.com, titled "Thoughts vs. Emotions," can help.

5. *Rating—Rate how strong your emotions are, from 1 to 10.* How powerful were the emotions you felt? Knowing how strong the emotions felt at the time of the situation can help you see which thoughts produce stronger emotions. It can also help you see how changing your thoughts can diminish those emotions.

Do This . . . Practice Using a Thought Record

Think of the situation I asked you to identify in step two's "Ponder This." Then, use the thought record in this book, or online to 1) hear your thoughts about the situation, 2) identify emotions, 3) tease them apart, and 4) write it all down. The example thought record, below, can show you how to do this. Give it a try now, but keep practicing for at least a week. Sometimes it takes even longer to begin to really get the hang of it, so give yourself as much time as you need.

Thought Record, Part 1 Example

Date	Situation Briefly Describe: *"What's going on?"*	Automatic Thought(s) *"What do I hear myself saying?"* *"What's going through my head?"* *"What sentences do I hear?"* Write your stream of automatic thoughts.	Emotion(s) *"What am I feeling?"* Identify/list emotions—sad, angry, frustrated . . . (There are usually more than one.)	Rate Rate the emotion, from 1-10. *"How powerful are my feelings?"*
Jan. 1	I was setting new year's goals and wanted to include exercising more.	"What's the point of even making a goal to exercise? You know you're not going to actually do it." "I never do what I say I'll do, especially when it comes to exercise." "I'm a failure, and I'll just fail again."	at first—motivated & then . . . frustrated down on myself afraid stressed depressed	9 10 9 6 10 8
Jan. 3	Went for a simple walk.	"I can't believe I'm actually doing this! Yay for me!" "I should really be running. Walking is too wimpy." "Whew. I can't breathe and my legs hurt after only a few minutes! I can't handle running. I knew I couldn't exercise. I'm such a wimp. I can't even handle a little jog! I'm such a loser!"	at first—excited, happy & then . . . insecure sad wimpy like a loser	10 9 10 9 10

Christina G. Hibbert, Psy.D. 2013
www.DrChristinaHibbert.com

Step 4: Challenge and Change
Unhealthy, Faulty, or Unhelpful Thoughts

Once you've got a full thought record, it's time to start making changes. In this step, we add the final two columns of the thought record, "rational or alternative response," and "outcome." The purpose is to 1) challenge irrational, unhealthy, or unhelpful thoughts, so you can then 2) change them into something more helpful, truthful, and rational.

Please note that these are difficult skills to master. Challenging thoughts can bring up emotions we didn't even know we had. It can shed light on experiences we didn't know even mattered. Go slowly and make sure you have support. Most of us will be practicing these skills for the rest of our lives (I know I still am!), so be patient with yourself, keep at it, and take breaks as needed.

Here's how:

1. *Identify irrational thoughts.* Look at your thought record and read through each of your "automatic thoughts." Ask, "Is this helpful? Is it truthful? Is it what I want?" Circle those that seem irrational, untruthful, or unhelpful.

2. *Use the "rational or alternative response" column to change your thoughts.* Look at each circled, irrational thought and ask yourself, "How can I make this more truthful, helpful, or rational?" For example, saying, "I can't go for a walk" is not true for most people. Most of us can walk. Instead, maybe you really mean, "I don't like walking," or maybe you mean, "I like walking, but I'm too tired today." Both of these are true and rational; you just have to find what works for you. Write your new thoughts in the "rational or alternative response" column.

3. *Use the "outcome" column to reevaluate your emotions.* How do you feel about the situation after finding the rational or alternative response? Re-rate how powerful each emotion is, from 1 to 10, using the "outcome" column. Often you'll find your emotions feel less strong after changing your thoughts.

Thought Record, Part 2

Date	Situation Briefly Describe: "What's going on?"	Automatic Thought(s) "What do I hear myself saying?" "What's going through my head?" "What sentences do I hear?" Write your stream of automatic thoughts.	Emotion(s) "What am I feeling?" 1. Identify/list emotions—sad, angry, frustrated . . . (There are usually more than one.) 2. Rate, 1-10	Alternative or Rational Response ("The Truth" or "Reality") "How else might I look at this?" "What is really happening?" Write an alternative to the automatic thoughts.	Outcome "How do I feel now?" Identify and rate emotions, 1-10, after the rational response.

Christina G. Hibbert, Psy.D. 2013
www.DrChristinaHibbert.com

If you're still unsure how to do this, the video demonstration, "Challenge and Change Thoughts Using a Thought Record" is available on my website, http://www.exercise4mentalhealth.com.

Do This . . . Challenge and Change Your Thoughts

After completing the "Do This" challenge from step three, apply the principles of step four to identify, challenge, and change unhealthy thoughts. Use the example thought record in this book or watch the video demonstrations at http://www.exercise4mentalhealth.com for help.

Step 5: Search for underlying themes, beliefs, or schema

After you've learned to hear your thoughts and separate them from your emotions, it's time to go back to your thought record and look for the themes, or beliefs, that underlie your thoughts and feelings. Cognitive-behavioral therapy calls these schema. Schema refers to the fundamental way we view ourselves, others, and the world. Our schema is, in essence, our worldview.

For example, many people have an underlying schema of "I'm not good enough." If we believe in our core that we're not good enough, it's going to interfere with our thinking, emotions, and behaviors. If I'm trying to begin a fitness class, become winded, and need to step out early, that schema of "I'm not good enough" is going to lead to thoughts like, "I knew I couldn't handle this. I'm an embarrassment. I can't do anything right." These thoughts will make me less likely to return to the class, and my belief that "I can't exercise" is once again affirmed.

If, however, I can identify the schema or belief—in this case, "I'm not good enough"—I can challenge it, investigate whether or not it's true, and gather evidence to create a new schema. Here's how:

1. *After completing several days of thought records, go back and examine the automatic thoughts, looking for common themes. For*

Thought Record, Part 2 Example

Date	Situation Briefly Describe: *"What's going on?"*	Automatic Thought(s) *"What do I hear myself saying?"* *"What's going through my head?"* *"What sentences do I hear?"* Write your stream of automatic thoughts.	Emotion(s) *"What am I feeling?"* 1. Identify/list emotions—sad, angry, frustrated.... (There are usually more than one.) 2. Rate, 1-10	Alternative or Rational Response ("The Truth" or "Reality") *"How else might I look at this?"* *"What is really happening?"* Write an alternative to the automatic thoughts.	Outcome *"How do I feel now?"* Identify and rate emotions, 1-10, after the rational response.
Jan. 1	I was setting new year's goals and wanted to include exercising more.	"What's the point of even making a goal to exercise? You know you're not going to actually do it." "I never do what I say I'll do, especially when it comes to exercise." "I'm a failure, and I'll just fail again."	motivated, 9 and then frustrated, 10 down on myself 9 afraid 6 stressed 10 depressed 8	"Just because I haven't been able to exercise regularly before doesn't mean I can't do it now." "I can do what I set my mind to, If I set specific, realistic goals for myself." "I'm not a failure. I just haven't figured out how to do this right—until now."	frustrated, 2 down on self 3 afraid 2 stressed 1 depressed 2
Jan. 3	Went for a simple walk.	"I can't believe I'm actually doing this! Yay for me!" "I should really be running. Walking is too wimpy." "Whew. I can't breathe and my legs hurt after only a few minutes! I can't handle running. I knew I couldn't exercise. I'm such a wimp. I can't even handle a little jog! I'm such a loser!"	excited, happy 10 and then insecure 8 sad 10 wimpy 10 like a loser 8	"I should feel proud that I'm beginning, even if I have to start slowly. Starting slowly is key to long-term success." "Walking is one of the best exercises, & I don't have to run to be 'strong,' or successful." "There's nothing wimpy about achieving my goals the right way."	excited, 5 happy, 5 insecure, 2 sad, 1 wimpy, 2 like a loser, 0

Christina G. Hibbert, Psy.D. 2013
www.DrChristinaHibbert.com

instance, you may see several thoughts that have a theme of "I'm not worthy," or perhaps, "I can't handle this," or "I'm not capable." See if you can find one or two common themes among the thoughts.

2. *Write down the schemas, underlying beliefs, or themes you discover.* Using the side, top, or back of the thought record, list any schemas you've found. For example, you may discover a schema that exercise is not going to benefit you, because "nothing good ever happens" to you, or that you can't achieve success because "you're not worthy of success." Once your schemas are identified and listed, you can begin to challenge them, just like you did in step four for your automatic thoughts.

3. *Using the same principles presented in step four, challenge each belief.* It can help to pretend you're investigating each belief, like a private detective. Question each one, asking, "Is this really true? What evidence do I have that this is true? What evidence do I have that this is not true?" Be honest and list as many ideas as you can.

4. *Go back through your evidence and see what you discover.* You may recognize that one list is much longer than another, you struggle to find evidence for one side or another, or it's clear your original schema was untrue. It can be tough to do this on your own, so I suggest involving a supportive person to help. A counselor is ideal, but a trusted friend, spouse/partner, or family member can help you sort through your beliefs and provide evidence that is honest, unbiased, and truthful.

For more help on how to challenge and change underlying schema, watch "Challenging and Changing Schema" at http://www.exercise4mentalhealth.com.

Reflection Questions: Schemas

1. What schemas, or underlying beliefs, about exercise for mental health did you discover when completing the suggestions in step five? List them all.

_____

_____

_____

_____

_____

_____

2. How might these schemas interfere with your exercise for mental health success?

_____

_____

_____

_____

_____

_____

3. If you could change these schemas in any way, how would you do so?

_____

_____

_____

_____

_____

_____

Step 6: When Unrealistic Thoughts/Beliefs Pop Up, Re-Affirm Your New Truths

Though positive affirmations can be a big help in overcoming unwanted thoughts and beliefs, much of the time, they don't work for one simple reason: we don't believe what we're saying to ourselves. I've seen this many times—clients who come in with a list of affirmations they got from some website, and then they confess they don't believe them at all. "I've been telling myself everyday in the mirror that 'I am strong,'" they say, "but I sure don't feel strong."

Affirmations only work if we believe them, and while it's possible to eventually believe the things we repeat in our mind, it's usually more helpful to affirm things we already know to be true. The word *affirm* means to remind oneself of something we already know. Instead of empty verbal affirmations, we must first discover the new thoughts, beliefs, and schemas that support our desires. We can then affirm these truths. Here's how:

1. *List your truthful affirmations.* Using the "rational or alternative thoughts" column as well as any of the new, truthful schemas you've created, list all the truths you've learned about exercise and mental health so far in your journal or digital device. You don't have to *feel* that they're true to have proven them to yourself, mentally. You may still feel weak when lifting weights, for instance, but once you've mentally proven weight lifting will eventually lead to you feeling stronger and more confident, it's tough to believe the automatic thoughts that say, "I can't do this," or "I'm weak." Instead, you can affirm what you already know by writing down, "I am strong, and as I continue my weight lifting, someday, I'll actually feel that strength."

2. *When untruthful automatic thoughts or beliefs arise, go to your list and select one or two truthful affirmations.* Repeat to yourself what you now know to be true. For example, if you're planning to exercise and hear the automatic thought, "I'm too tired," go to your list and pick a truth to affirm in your mind. Perhaps say, "If I go for a jog, I'll feel more energized," or "If I do yoga, I'll feel less stiff and sore, and more relaxed and ready for the day." Affirming truths is an effective way to make change not only in how we think, but also in how we feel, how our body feels, and what we do.

Truthful Affirmations for Mental Health Through Exercise

Some helpful truthful affirmations, when it comes to exercise for mental health, include:

- "When my mood is off, I should take a walk. I know it will give me the boost I need to turn the day around."

- "I know lifting weights will help me feel less tense in my body, even though I feel so anxious right now."
- "Even though I'm stressed, I know if I exercise I'll be so much better able to handle the day."
- "Even though I'm feeling depressed today, I know I need to exercise. It will clear the clouds from my mind and getting out into the sun will help as well."

Do the work in the six steps above so you can discover the truths that work for you. You have to believe them to achieve them; then, reaffirm them as often as needed.

Reflection Questions:
Exercise for Mental Health Affirmations

1. Using the steps above, identify and list five truthful exercise for mental health affirmations. Remember, you don't have to completely feel the truth of them yet; you simply have to believe in them.

_____

_____

_____

_____

_____

_____

_____

_____

2. Post your affirmations where you'll see them often. When thoughts start to drag you down, go to your list and remind yourself of what you know to be true. Let it help you be motivated and overcome the roadblocks you face.

We Can Change

Now, back to Tammy and Matt. As we worked on the steps of change, presented above, Tammy and Matt used thought records to identify and challenge their unhealthy beliefs. Tammy worked to understand and build her self-worth by keeping track of her self-defeating thoughts and challenging them. She began to see for herself her schema of "I'm inadequate," and only then could she begin to make change. She also began to incorporate exercise into her daily routine, using her thought record to identify blocks that prevented her from sticking to her goals.

Matt has worked hard to understand his resentments, and using the thought record, he began to see just how deeply they ran. He's been working through them, learning to trust his wife again, and the couple has used the thought records to share what they're realizing, reconnect, and understand one another better. Matt has started joining Tammy in exercise. Since Tammy was a collegiate tennis player, they set up a court in their backyard and play most days, as a family or couple. "We go out in the backyard when we have a problem and whack the ball back and forth while we work it out," they say. Working out together is helping them work things out.

We can change our feelings about exercise; we can change our thoughts, beliefs, and schemas. In doing so, we can change the way we approach exercise, our ability to stick with exercise, and yes, we can positively change our physical and mental health. It takes work. It takes time and effort and a desire to change. It takes learning the skills presented above and actively applying them in our life. But, with time, effort, and desire, we can work through that spiral of change and one day find ourselves in maintenance mode, basking in the many gifts exercise has to offer.

KEY 6

OVERCOME ROADBLOCKS

"There are plenty of difficult obstacles in your path. Don't allow yourself to become one of them."

—Ralph Marston

It's true. There are plenty of difficult obstacles when it comes to exercise for mental health. Some roadblocks are physical, like illness, injury, or bodily reactions to exercise. Others are mental, like feeling too depressed, unmotivated, or self-conscious to exercise. Some may even be both mental and physical, like getting so anxious when you exercise that it creates the physical sensation of panic, stopping you in your tracks. All can present very real challenges to beginning, persisting in, and adhering to all types of physical activity.

It's also true that we can overcome these roadblocks. That's what this key is all about. Challenges are part of life, in every aspect, and, as I wrote in *This is How We Grow*, "...we can *go* through them, or we can choose to *grow* through them" (2013, p. 414). When we choose to exercise to improve our mental health and emotional, social, and spiritual well-being, we are choosing to grow. That's what we're here for—to take life's challenges, identify the roadblocks, and either to remove them from our path or find a way around them.

As we just worked on in Key 5, we can identify, question, and find alternative responses to the roadblocks we face. Many times we feel like we're the only one facing the particular things that block our exercise for mental health potential, but most roadblocks are quite common, and there are some excellent, specific strategies we can employ to break through and leave them in the dust.

Physical and Mental Fortitude in Overcoming Roadblocks

Most of us tend to focus on how physically challenging exercise can be. However, while it can certainly present physical challenges, exercise requires just as much, if not more, mental fortitude. Even if our main roadblock is physical, like dealing with a chronic illness, it still comes back to our thoughts and motivations about exercise. For instance, we can choose to quit exercising altogether, or we can work with our doctor to see what types of exercise might benefit us most. We can stay motivated even when we face roadblocks. We can find a way to overcome them. We can choose to grow.

It helps to be mentally strong if we want to become physically strong. That's why we've been focusing on building motivation, setting goals, understanding change, and learning how to tackle unhelpful thoughts in keys 4 and 5, before I've actually asked you to start exercising. This is an important point, and one that most of us often miss: *being mentally prepared to exercise is just as important as doing the physical work of exercise.* In fact, without mental awareness, skill building, and fortitude, our chances of exercise success are slim.

If you're reading this and saying, "Great. I have no mental fortitude. I guess I'm a lost cause," my reply is, "Wrong!" Mental fortitude is a skill we can develop, improve, and build. Like any other skill, from learning to play an instrument to knowing how to fix a car, it takes learning, time, and practice, practice, practice. Hopefully, as you've been reading through keys 4 and 5, you've come to see this for yourself: you can change your mental outlook and approaches to exercise, mental health, and life—if you're willing to work.

Hopefully, you've already started doing the work I've suggested in each key. Now, let's apply the ideas, methods, and skills you've been working on by taking a deeper look into the specific challenges we all face when it comes to exercise for mental health. Then, we can build our mental fortitude to overcome them.

Common Roadblocks to Exercise and How to Overcome Them

As we go through the long list of potential blocks to exercise for mental health success, pay attention to those with which you most identify. Perhaps you might place a little mark next to those that are relevant, or make a mental note. Pay close attention to the strategies outlined for overcoming these particular roadblocks, and ponder which feel most helpful. We'll discuss your reactions in more detail at the end of this key.

The most common roadblocks to exercise for mental health include the following:

Time and Responsibilities

"I don't have time to exercise."
This is probably the most popular excuse when it comes to exercise, and it is an excuse. Yes, life is busy, especially in today's world, and yes, many days it can feel like we have no time for exercise. Some days that may even be true. But for most of us, if we really get honest, we know deep down that if we prioritized exercise, then we would make the time, right? Here's how:

- *Identify your priorities, and cut those that are least important.* What matters most to you? If mental health is on your list, then exercise needs to be, too. Years ago, when I had young children, was in graduate school, working part-time, and finishing my dissertation, all while my husband was in dental school, I found myself depressed and overwhelmed. One day, I decided to list my priorities. My list included my children and husband, faith and spiritual connection, doing my best in school, and keeping myself mentally and physically healthy. Knowing these priorities helped me examine my weekly schedule and cut what wasn't a priority. This, in turn, allowed me to use that time to exercise, get enough sleep, and get some much-needed alone time. All of these things keep me mentally healthy. It all comes back to setting—and honoring—priorities.

- *Plan and schedule exercise.* Don't just wait until you wake up to decide if you'll exercise that day. Sit down and carve out realistic blocks of time for exercise, and put them in your weekly schedule.

- *Exercise early in the day.* Seek to do your top priorities first. If you have to go to work early, then schedule exercise for later, but try to get to it as early in the day as possible. This makes it more likely you'll do it, even when it feels like you don't have time.

- *Incorporate exercise into activities you already do.* If you have to drive the kids to after-school events, stay and go for a walk instead of heading home and coming back. When cleaning the house, try to keep moving for 20 minutes straight, to raise your heart rate and experience the payoff. The more you add movement to what you're already doing, the more time you save.

"I'm too busy. I work all day, and when I get home, my family needs me."

Work is often quoted as a major reason people don't exercise. "I'm too busy." "Work is too stressful." "When I get home, I only have time for my family, or I'm too exhausted." It's certainly difficult to balance work, home, and family life, not to mention adding in exercise.

For many, the work-home balance is a huge factor in the level of perceived life stress, and consequently, in how much you exercise. However, research also shows that exercise may be just what you need. Studies show a clear relationship between exercise and one's ability to manage work and home. Intuitively, it seems that exercising presents just one more "thing to do" when time is already scarce, and this is precisely why so many parents and working professionals drop it. Yet, because exercise reduces stress, it provides a release that enables greater work productivity and family interaction. As one researcher put it, "A reduction in stress is tantamount to an expansion of time" (Clayton 2014).

Eric, 40, is an orthodontist and married father of two. He's been active his whole life and has found a way to stay active, despite growing responsibilities as a father and business owner. "I love being active, especially outdoors," Eric says. "But I don't want to miss quality time with my family. So, I run early in the morning, or sometimes, when training, in the night, when my family's asleep." This way, Eric doesn't impinge on family or worktime, yet still reaps the benefits of exercise that he loves, including feeling more present, at work and at home. "Physical activity clears the mind," he says, "whatever is on the plate."

Here are some ways to better incorporate time for exercise for mental health into an already packed schedule:

- *Add activity into your workday.* Every 30 minutes, stand and stretch, march in place, or walk around the office. Take walking breaks, or plan a walking meeting. Use your lunch break to hit the gym or take a walk. It will not only add physical activity into your day, but it will also reduce bodily tension and relieve stress.
- *Use family time for exercise.* As we demonstrated in Key 3, exercising as a family is a win-win-win. You and your family members get the movement your minds and bodies need, quality, fun family time, and you save time by doing it all at the same time. You're building relationships and mental health all at once.
- *Remind yourself how much exercise will help.* Like Eric said above, if you can remind yourself of the benefits of exercise, even when time is limited, you will fit it in. "I always feel better after hitting the gym on my way home," or "The stress will melt away if I can just take the dog out for a walk." These things remind you it's worth the effort to make it happen.
- *Take a walk with your partner/spouse after a long day and talk about your day.* Not only is this a good way to de-stress your body

and mind, but it's also a great way to build the connection between you and your partner and get you on the same page.

"I have too many family responsibilities to exercise!"

Family responsibilities can seem endless, especially when you're on duty as mom or dad, 24/7. Babies and young children can make it tough to get away, and older kids can have relentless schedules with which you're simply trying to keep up.

It is possible to maintain a regular exercise program with babies, young children, teens, and at all stages of family life. With six kids of my own, trust me, I know. The good news is that developing an exercise program now will not only benefit your physical and mental health; it will also benefit your children.

In addition to the tips in Key 3 on exercising with your family, here are a few other things you can try:

- *Monitor your activities for one week.* Identify at least three, 30-minute time periods you can carve out for exercise. Then, use them to do activities that are simple and don't require transportation—like climbing stairs in your home, taking laps around your neighborhood, or doing simple body strengthening moves like push-ups, sit-ups, or squats, to music in your living room.

- *Involve your baby in your exercise program.* Put baby in a front-pack and do squats or lunges. Place her in a bouncer and do a kickboxing video, making faces and interacting with her while you do. Use a stroller or sling and go for a walk; research shows that stroller, or pram, walking is an excellent way to improve mental health with your baby.

- *Create a home exercise studio and exercise during naptime.* This can help you cut your exercise time, and it doesn't have to cost a lot of money either. Purchase a couple dumbbells, some favorite DVDs, and a yoga mat, to start. During naps, head to your exercise area and do a home video, lift free weights, or stretch.

- *Join a gym with babysitting included or trade off babysitting.* I taught aerobics for years using the free babysitting, and my kids loved getting to play while I worked out. If you're not the gym type, then alternate babysitting with a friend so you can exercise. Couples can take turns with one another, watching the kids while the other exercises.

- *Involve friends.* Meet at the park and take turns watching the kids while the other goes for a jog, or start a babysitting co-op, where each person takes a turn watching all the children, and rotate.
- *Little kids can exercise with you.* When my kids were very young, they used to stretch and attempt yoga with me, or they'd ride their Big Wheel up and down the street, while I ran alongside. It's a great way to instill in kids a love of exercise, too.
- *Older kids and teens can workout with you, too.* As kids get older, invite them to join your home workout or take them to the gym with you. Teach them how to safely lift weights, do cardio, or use the machines. It's great bonding time and you're also teaching them important skills they'll use their whole lives.
- *Be active with your kids.* Play tag, keep away, or other running games. Challenge each other to an activity-based video game, or use an app like Sworkit, where kids can select a time limit and type of activity and then complete exercise challenges to fit their needs. Doing things together makes everything more fun, and doable.

"I never have the same block of time to exercise each day, so it's tough to plan."

You don't need to exercise at a consistent time of day; you just need to exercise consistently. And you don't have to exercise in one solid block to get the benefits of exercise for mental health, either. Just move, attempting to total at least 30 minutes, three or more times a week, whenever you can fit it in.

These strategies will help:

- *Break up exercise as needed.* Perhaps start with two, 10-minute blocks of exercise, before work and on a break. Or try 15 minutes in the morning and 15 minutes after dinner.
- *Take mini exercise breaks throughout the day.* Get creative. At home, take continuous breaks to do a few planks, pull-ups, or

twists, even for a few minutes at a time. At work, take mini exercise breaks every hour or so. If you can, get together with coworkers and do jumping jacks, squats, or stair climbing. Or, sit on the floor during a meeting so everyone can stretch. You'd be surprised how much these mini breaks can add up.

"I plan on exercising after work, but something always seems to come up, or I have to stay late."

Hey, it happens, and it's okay. As mentioned earlier, whenever possible, try to schedule your exercise for first thing in the morning. If this isn't possible, find another way to keep your commitment to exercise, even if it's the next morning or afternoon.

Here are some tips for making this happen:

- Call a friend and set a date to take a brisk walk before work the next day.
- Keep your exercise clothes and shoes with you at all times, so if you end up with free time or a break in the next day or two, you can make up the exercise then.

Low Motivation, Boredom, and Fatigue

"I don't feel motivated."

As we discussed at length in Key 4, it's hard to start and stick with an exercise program when we don't feel motivated. Notice the key word there—no, not *motivation*—*feel*. Motivation is all about how we feel. We think, "I want to exercise because I know it will help me feel mentally and physically healthy and happy," but we *feel* tired, stressed, or low energy—unmotivated.

When it comes to exercise for mental health, there are internal motivators and external motivators, as we outlined in Key 4. We are most likely to stick with exercise when motivated by both. External motivators to exercise include things like: a mental health diagnosis, like depression or anxiety; a physical health diagnosis, like type two diabetes, cancer, or fibromyalgia; or comparing ourselves to others. Many people start exercising because of these types of external factors, which is a good thing, of course, since it gets them moving. The trouble is it's challenging to maintain motivation unless we also discover and increase our internal motivators.

Internal motivation begins with our beliefs about exercise.

Ponder This . . .

Do you believe you need exercise in your life? Do you believe you will receive the benefits we discussed in part one by exercising regularly? Do you believe you can and will stick with it?

These, and other questions like these, can help you determine what you really think about exercise and your motivation to do it. By examining these questions you can work to increase your internal motivation. Common internal motivators include: loving yourself and your family, a desire for improved mental health, a desire for increased happiness, and a drive to embrace your self-worth and develop the self-confidence to know that you can, and will, achieve your goals.

For example, if you believe you will feel mentally healthy if you exercise, or if you believe you and your family will benefit from it, you're much more likely to stick with your exercise routine. "I'm doing this for my family, and for myself," is a powerful internal motivator. Other beliefs like, "I know I'll feel so much happier today if I get up and exercise," have a similarly powerful effect.

I call this "discovering your *why*." Why do you want to exercise? What motivates you? Identifying your internal *why* is a powerful way to stay motivated. If your *why* is a love of mental and spiritual wellness, it can lead you to engage in more relaxing exercises; whereas, if your *why* is increasing energy and happiness, you may want more cardiovascular exercise. We may have more than one *why* that drives us, or only one. The most important thing is to take the time to identify what your *why* is and remind yourself of it when you need a motivation boost.

Reflection Questions: Discover Your Why

1. Take a few minutes to get still and comfortable. Close your eyes, take a deep breath, and sit calmly. Ponder this question: "What is my *why* for exercise?" It's important to identify our *why* if we want to fulfill it. What is your *why*?

   _____

   _____

   _____

   _____

   _____

2. What internal beliefs/values motivate you to exercise?

   _____

   _____

   _____

   _____

   _____

3. What internal beliefs/values motivate you to take charge of your mental health and well-being?

   _____

   _____

   _____

   _____

   _____

Along with building motivation, we can also work on overcoming un-motivation.

When we feel unmotivated, it can be difficult to do much of anything. This is one of the many things that makes depression so hard. A key element of depression is that it zaps motivation, energy, and drive, making it feel much harder than normal to do even the simplest things. Ironically, exercise—one of the best things you can do to feel less depressed—is often the last thing you feel like doing. The same goes for other reasons we may be unmotivated, like feeling too tired, stressed, or anxious—exercise is a cure for each of these, but first we have to get ourselves up and moving. How?

- *Start small.* Tell yourself, "I'm just going to get up and walk outside to get the mail." Then, once you're at the mailbox, you may decide to walk to the corner and back. Or, you might not, but at least you got yourself up and out the door. Eventually, you may decide to walk around the block, and by then you may have enough energy to come back and do some sit-ups and then stretch. This is an incredibly helpful concept: give yourself small goals, and then add to them as you see fit. "I'm just going to put on my workout clothes;" "I'll just march in place during one commercial break;" "I just have to do five minutes of my yoga video." Doing these things will likely develop into actually working out in those workout clothes, marching in place during all the commercial breaks, and doing the full yoga video. Start small and go from there.
- *Exercise at the right time of day, on the right days of the week.* When do you feel most energized? I'm a morning person, so I know I'm more motivated to exercise first thing in the morning than later in the day. Perhaps you're a night owl, and playing baseball with your kids after dinner is going to be when you feel most energized. The same goes for the days of the week. Exercise may always be tougher to fit in on certain days. For instance, I find that I'm much better at exercising on school days than on weekends, when there's no routine and all my kids are home, needing my full attention. So, I exercise weekday mornings, and then on Saturdays, I try to fit in a family activity. I take Sundays off. Others will find the weekends are ideal and weekdays are tougher. Whenever you'll have the best chance for success, plan your exercise around that.
- *Plan exercise on your calendar and then check it off.* Schedule exercise or physical activities just like you would any other important appointment, then "check it off" when it's complete. Having that moment of checking it off can be a huge motivator.

- *Go slowly.* One of the biggest factors influencing exercise motivation is trying to do too much too soon. We get excited to start, so we start with a bang. But soon, we feel overwhelmed, exhausted, and unable to keep up with the goals we've set. Starting slowly and building your exercise routine, bit by bit, is key to staying motivated, long-term.

"I'm too tired."

Life is tiring, and this can be a huge reason many of us fail to exercise. We're just too darn exhausted to get up and do it. However, exercising when we're tired, especially doing mild cardiovascular exercise like walking, is actually one of the best things we can do to perk up. It increases energy faster than pretty much any other solution, and gives lasting energy to get through the rest of the day.

Here are some ways to overcome being too tired to exercise:

- *Exercise first thing in the morning.* We tend to be freshest just after we wake up, and exercising first thing also helps keep us awake and alert throughout the day.
- *Give yourself a short exercise challenge.* Tell yourself you'll do 10 minutes, and then, if you're still feeling too tired, you can stop. Chances are, you'll feel up to "just five more."
- *Remind yourself how getting up and moving will increase your energy.* When I feel sluggish in the afternoon, I remind myself I usually need either a power nap or a brisk walk. Once you feel the effects of exercise on your energy, remind yourself of this, every day if needed.
- *Remember the connection between exercise and sleep.* If you're tired because you're not getting enough sleep, then remember how exercise and sleep interplay. If you can get more sleep, you'll feel better able to exercise, and if you exercise, you'll sleep better.

"Exercise is boring."

The reason exercise feels boring is because we tell ourselves we have to run, or do push-ups, or take a spinning class, when we don't enjoy any of those things. True, we may learn to enjoy them as we experience the payoffs of exercise, but there are also such a variety of ways to exercise that it's good to step out of our "box" and mix it up.

Also, remember that you don't have to "workout" to exercise. Exercise for mental health is about moving, being active, and as much as possible, having fun.

Here are a few tips to help you beat the boredom:

- *Choose activities you actually enjoy rather than forcing yourself to do exercises you can't stand.* If you're not fond of fitness classes, that's okay. You can dance at home, roller skate, swim, or garden instead. If you're doing something you enjoy, you're much more likely to keep doing it.
- *Incorporate an activity you enjoy into your existing routine.* Watch TV while you stretch, get out and move while talking with a friend, bring your tablet and play games, or read while you're on the treadmill. Incorporating activities you enjoy into physical activity helps make it more interesting and fun.
- *Try something completely new.* Brand new activities keep exercise fresh for our brains and muscles. I remember the first time I tried Pilates, with a home exercise video. The next day, I felt it—sore in muscles I didn't know existed—but Pilates was so new and intriguing to me that I couldn't wait to do it again. What new activities might you like to try? Put one on your calendar for this week, and then keep trying until you find something that holds your interest. (We'll talk more about "good" versus "bad" sore, below.)

Nan struggled with exercise after she left high school and her "sports days" behind. When younger, she didn't have to think about exercise because she was always active in softball and volleyball. As she moved on to college, career, and marriage, she began to feel more overwhelmed, stressed, and eventually depressed. She wanted to exercise, but nothing appealed to her. The sports she used to enjoy didn't hold the same thrill now that she wasn't on a team with friends. Even though she had older sisters who worked out regularly and with whom she could exercise, Nan could never get into it like they did. She'd tried walking, jogging, running, and swimming, like her sisters, but they just didn't interest Nan enough for her to stick with them.

Until she discovered Zumba, a dance/exercise hybrid. A friend recommended it, and at first she didn't even want to try it. "What was the point?" she thought. She felt self-conscious the first time, especially since she felt out of shape and had never tried Zumba before, but going with her friend helped, and the teacher made her comfortable by emphasizing fun and encouraging the group not to worry if they didn't get the moves just right. Not only was Zumba fun and engaging, it kept her mind off the fact that she was exercising. It provided built-in social support, not just with the friend who invited her, but new friends she made in class. "Zumba has made being active fun again," Nan says. And as she's committed to her Zumba classes, she's experienced less stress and fewer depressed days. She's also improved her nutrition and consequently lost 50 pounds. "I wasn't focused on weight loss or 'exercising,'" Nan says. "I was focused on feeling better by finding a way to make being active fun. I found it, and it happened to get me in shape, too." She also reports she's finding greater self-confidence as she stays with it—a definite bonus.

Mental and Emotional Concerns

"I'm too stressed."

Life's stress can definitely make it hard to get out and exercise. Work, family, finances, health, commitments, and responsibilities—it can all feel like too much, for everyone, at times. However, when we feel too stressed to exercise is probably when we need it most. Exercise calms us, boosts our mood, and relieves tension, reducing overall stress. And in today's too-busy world, most of us desperately need a little stress reduction. (See Key 1 for more of the benefits of exercise on stress.)

Stress is associated with many negative consequences in the body and mind. In the body, stress can lead to aches, pains, sleeplessness, acne, poor eating habits, unhealthy weight gain/loss, back/neck problems, irritable bowel syndrome (IBS), headaches, increased risk for cancer, illness, heart problems, and so on. In the mind, stress is associated with burnout, depression, anxiety, anger, irritability, low self-worth, and is a contributing factor or trigger for most other mental and emotional disorders. Bottom line: stress is no good.

Short-term stress is bad enough, but prolonged stress can do major damage. We're not made to stay in that heightened state of alarm stress puts us in—in the fight-or-flight state, where our body is bathing in the stress hormone, cortisol. Cortisol has been called "public enemy number one," since it is associated with increased risk for depression and mental illness, poorer learning and memory, decreased immune function, heart disease, and even lower life expectancy, to name a few (Bergland, 2013). Because of this, chronic stress can not only make existing mental and physical conditions worse, but can lead to serious physical and mental health issues.

When we limit stressors, we will feel less stressed, but there are many stressors (like kids, work, or caregiving) than can't be removed. Thus, the key to stress management is really to 1) remove the stressors we can, and 2) manage our responses to the stressors we cannot. Exercise is one of the best ways to do this. Here are some suggestions for how:

- *Combine physical activity with stress reduction and relaxation.* Yoga, Pilates, Tai Chi, or stretching can be quite relaxing while also giving you the mental health benefits of exercise—and they're excellent stress-relievers. Going for an easy walk with a friend while you vent your stress combines movement with the added benefit of social engagement and processing.
- *Practice mindfulness/breathing/gratitude/meditation/prayer while you move.* Each of these practices has been shown to reduce overall stress and help quiet your mind. Combining them with exercise, which also reduces stress and calms your mind, is a double-whammy of stress reduction. Practice walking meditation, take a hike and focus on nature, think of all you're grateful for as you bike ride, or pray while stretching.

- *Try an "hour of power."* Exercise can become part of a daily, centering, stress reduction plan. Several years ago, I started doing a morning "hour of power," which, for me, involves 30 minutes of walking or jogging while I focus on nature, breathing, and gratitude, followed by 30 minutes of stretching and meditation, scripture study, and prayer. When I get out of the habit of doing this, I immediately feel more tension and stress in my daily life. What would your "hour of power" contain? Try it out. It's an excellent way to start each day and prevent, or reduce, stress.
- *If your body is feeling the effects of stress, try weight-lifting.* If you're experiencing muscle tension as a result of stress, then lifting light to medium weights is a great solution. It works your muscles, which actually moves and stretches them. It also increases blood flow, which makes muscles less sore and helps you feel calmer and more energized. And remember, ladies, weight lifting isn't just for the guys, and isn't just for making big muscles. It also increases bone density, which helps fight osteoporosis, and is a great way to tone up. (See Key 7 for more on weight lifting and strength training.)
- *Turn exercise into play.* Most adults fail miserably at this one, yet play researcher Stuart Brown has said, "The opposite of play is not work. The opposite of play is depression" (2008). We need play—time without purpose, time when we forget our stresses or how we're perceived, time we want to last. What physical activities light you up? What makes you feel young and engaged with life? Is it throwing a ball around with your kids, jumping on a trampoline, playing flag football with friends, golfing, or playing water basketball as a family? Make exercise a time for play. You'll feel less stressed, save time, and probably fall asleep a little happier, too.

"I am too overcome by my feelings to exercise."

Situations of loss, heartache, or mental illness like depression, anxiety, and so forth, usually carry with them intense emotions that can feel overwhelming. Feelings like sadness, pain, grief, worry, or fear can overtake us, leaving us paralyzed and unable to do much of anything, let alone exercise. Exercise can help us process power-ful emotions. Remember Mechelle's story, from Key 1? As she made herself walk, and then run, she was able to use exercise to work through extreme pain, grief, sadness, and fear. You can do the same.

On the flip side, as you work on processing and feeling your emotions, you will feel more able to motivate yourself to exercise. Hard as it may sound, the way to heal from emotional pain is to feel the emotional pain. "To me, FEEL means Freely Experience Emotions with Love" (Hibbert, 2013). As we FEEL the powerful emotions that come, we begin to see they are not as powerful as we think. Feelings lose their power as we sit with them and lovingly let them be.

How do we FEEL? First, sit in a comfortable, quiet place. Close your eyes, and breathe deeply. As you breathe, let the emotions come. Whatever they may be—fear, heartache, disappoint-ment, grief, sadness, worry, pain—just let them be. Continue to breathe through the emotions like you would if you were experi-encing physical pain. Then, imagine yourself "leaning back" from the emotions. As you lean back, the feelings stay in front of you. You can still feel them, but you now see that these emotions are not part of you. They're just feelings, not you. Do this activity for a couple of minutes, until you feel the emotion release or until you need a break. Repeat each day until the emotions begin to dissipate. If you have extremely painful or overwhelming emo-tions that are significantly impacting your daily life, then seek help from a mental health professional. (For a video demonstra-tion of how to FEEL, watch "How to FEEL Powerful Emotions," at http://www.exercise4mentalhealth.com.)

The best-case scenario is to process our intense emotions while also incorporating exercise into each day. Use FEEL to practice getting a grip on powerful emotions. Then, try these ideas, too:

- *Do a calming exercise practice.* Exercises that are meditative, focus on breathing, or incorporate mindfulness can help calm powerful emotions.

- *Take an exercise class.* Exercising with others can get your mind off your emotions while also giving you a built-in support system for when you need to talk.
- *Exercise in nature.* Get out into beautiful, still places when you exercise. Stop and take some time to FEEL. Then, get up and get going again.
- *Revisit your exercise affirmations.* Be sure to include an affirmation that "If I move my body, it will move these emotions." It's true. Moving the body does help free intense emotions. Remind yourself of this as often as you need.

"I'm too immobilized by depression to exercise."
Depressed clients routinely tell me that they know exercise would help, but they just can't seem to make themselves get up and begin. As I mentioned above, depression can zap motivation, energy, and drive, making it feel impossible to get out and exercise. The tools for motivation and thought-changing in keys 4 and 5 can help, and I encourage all who suffer from depression to make a concerted effort to learn and practice those skills. In extreme cases, if your depression is truly insurmountable, an immoveable obstacle, work with your doctor to focus on alleviating symptoms to the point where exercise becomes possible again. (*See note about mental illness at the end of this passage.)

Additionally, try these things:

- *Enlist an exercise buddy.* When you're struggling with depression, this is one of the best things you can do. Partner with someone who will show up, inspire you to get up, and hold you to your commitment to exercise. When you feel accountable to someone else it can force you to get out the door even when you'd much rather stay home. It has the added benefit of helping you connect with others, thus challenging the urge to remain isolated.
- *Take it slow and easy.* You don't need to move quickly, or for a very long time period, or make the movement challenging. With depression, your goal is simply to move. Plain old walking—not

jogging or running or even brisk walking—for even 10 minutes at a time, is a good place to start with depression.

- *Make walking part of your regular schedule and part of your treatment plan.* Because walking is so good for your mood, brain, body, and spirit, create a routine that includes a daily walk. Start slow and easy, and then add time to your walk as you feel stronger.

- *Get outside.* Sunlight therapy is an effective treatment for depression, and when you add sunlight to movement, you get a double dose. If you're able to be in a beautiful place while you exercise, all the better. Nature has a way of lifting the spirits the same way sunshine and exercise do.

"Exercise makes me too anxious. I feel like I'm having a panic attack."

This is a very real problem for many, especially for those who suffer from anxiety disorders of all types, including phobias, OCD, PTSD, and especially panic disorder. Anxiety and panic involve hyper-arousal, meaning the fear or worry the person experiences becomes so intense that it manifests physically—in an increased heart rate, a shot of adrenaline, and quick, shallow breathing. Since exercise produces similar sensations—an increased heart rate, boost in adrenaline, and quick, shallow breathing—many suffering from anxiety feel more anxious, fearful, or worried when they exercise. In a very real way, exercise can feel like, or even turn into, a panic attack, which can then generate greater fear or anxiety. Exercise, for many, is too reminiscent of the anxiety they're seeking to overcome through exercise. It can be a vicious cycle.

Case example: Summer had lived with anxiety and panic attacks for years and had long heard about the many benefits of exercise for anxiety (we learned all about these in Key 1). She believed what she heard from friends, family, and doctors—that exercise could reduce her anxiety, lower her stress, help her sleep better, and even calm the heart palpitations she'd been experiencing as part of her anxiety disorder—but it took a significant length of time before she gave it a try.

Finally, one day, feeling anxious about an upcoming test in her graduate school program, she said, "I decided to take everyone's advice and expose myself to the miracle cure that is exercise." She walked down to the conveniently located gym in her apartment complex, got on an elliptical machine, and had a panic attack. "And I never went back," she said. Summer became afraid of exercise—afraid of how it felt and afraid that if she tried it again it would only cause her more panic.

Summer, who is a mental health professional, knew her fears were irrational. Having studied CBT, she knew her thoughts were faulty. Having studied health, she knew the increased heart rate from exercise actually strengthened her heart and was good for her. But it took some time for Summer to figure out how to get over her fears.

Eventually, Summer did overcome her fears, and she had the foresight to take good notes on what helped her so she can now help others do the same (Beretsky, 2011). Below, I've combined some of Summer's suggestions for overcoming exercise anxiety and panic with my own:

- *Begin in an environment that's comfortable.* Start at home or wherever you feel most relaxed. Forget about the gym for now, especially if it might trigger symptoms.
- *Select activities that are relaxing or fun.* Don't start by running on a treadmill or doing jumping jacks. Try something that is more calming, like a Tai Chi video on YouTube, stretching outside in the morning, or something you enjoy, like easy hiking with your friends. Again, your goal isn't necessarily to "workout." It's to move, and do so in as comfortable a way as possible.
- *Start with small steps.* It doesn't matter how small the steps or how long it takes to take larger steps; what matters is you're taking steps. Summer suggests that you start with very small steps, like 30 seconds of dancing on day one. "Then, stop. Don't overdo it on the first day. Try a full minute on day two. If that works, try two minutes the next day. Such a gentle schedule might sound laughable, sure, but don't let anyone tell you that you ought to be doing more right away. The goal, at this point, is to reacquaint yourself with the

physical sensations of exercise. Two minutes of dancing around in your apartment is better than nothing" (Beretsky, 2011).

- *At first, distract yourself from the sensations of exercise.* It helps, when starting, to distract yourself from how you feel when you exercise, through TV, music, reading, listening to a podcast, or anything to take your mind off how your body feels.

- *Slowly expose yourself to the sensations of exercise in other settings.* This is part of exposure therapy, which is the recommended treatment for panic disorder and anxiety. Exposing yourself to situations that elicit similar bodily sensations as exercise but are less threatening can help you adjust to your body's responses. For example, Summer suggests that if sweating triggers feelings of panic in you, then you might remain in the bathroom after a hot shower and let yourself feel the moisture and sweat on your skin and body (Beretsky, 2011). Over time, doing these types of exposure experiences helps you feel less triggered and more able to accept them during exercise.

- *Practice self-love.* We talked about self-love in Key 3, and this is a perfect place to practice it. Before doing the things suggested above, take a few moments to breathe and remember your *why* (see above). Remind yourself you're doing this because you love yourself, want to be kind to yourself, and give yourself the best mental and physical health possible. Then, love yourself through these suggestions. Love yourself by beginning. Love yourself by stopping when you need to. Love yourself by beginning again tomorrow. Acknowledge every little step you take, and let yourself feel accomplished.

*Note About Mental Illness: *At times, those who struggle with mental illness will be so overcome by their symptoms that exercise isn't feasible. If you're experiencing severe symptoms of any mental health disorder, please seek help from your medical and mental health providers to stabilize you, first. Then, seek their advice about how to incorporate exercise into your treatment plan.*

Physical Health Concerns

"It hurts when I exercise."

The idea of "no pain, no gain," is not a healthy one. Exercise shouldn't be painful. Yes, you might be pushing yourself, and yes, you might feel a bit sore, especially if you're doing an activity for the first time, but pain should not be part of your exercise routine.

First, it's important to understand what *hurt* means to you. *Hurt* may mean uncomfortable—out of breath and sore, especially the next day. Or, *hurt* may be pain, injury, or illness. You shouldn't feel pain when you exercise, and you shouldn't feel sick either. Remember Julie, from Key 3? Nausea and vomiting are not part of a healthy exercise routine, and if you continue exercising when in pain or ill, it can cause injury or further illness.

There's a difference between "good sore" and "bad sore." "Good sore" is the feeling you have the day after a good, hard workout, when you've tried something new, involved muscles you don't typically utilize, or have used your body in a new way. When you're "good sore," you can still move and you're not in pain, though you will definitely want to refrain from working those muscles for a few days, to let them recover.

"Bad sore" means you're pushing your body too far. Breathing too heavily, stretching muscles so far they cause pain, or pushing yourself so hard you injure your body are all indications that what you're doing is not healthy. Exercise should heal the body, not wreck it. It's important to be mindful of these distinctions in order to prevent pain, injuries, and even illness from exercise.

That being said, it's also okay to feel a little uncomfortable when exercising, especially at first, or to push yourself just enough to feel "good sore" when you're done. Here are a few strategies to help you out:

- *Choose a simple activity you know you can safely do.* Choose something like plain and simple walking (always the go-to exercise). The more you practice, the more you'll build skills and eventually you can add other activities, more time, or more intensity to your exercise routine. Whether you're starting exercise for the first time ever or re-starting after a significant break, it's important to start slowly.

- *Try an exercise class that's just for beginners, or work with a personal trainer.* A good instructor will explain how to prevent injury, monitor you, and provide feedback to help you improve safely. Having someone guide you through the exercise process and teach safety procedures is very helpful, especially when you're new to exercise.

- *If you're recovering from an injury, try physical therapy.* A physical therapist can help you move your body in a safe and effective way to get you back to where you want your body to be.

- *If you're feeling uncomfortable during exercise (but aren't experiencing pain), then focus on something else to distract you from your body.* If lifting weights, focus on counting reps or increasing your range of motion. If doing cardio on a machine at the gym after work, watch the news, people-watch, or flip through a magazine to keep your mind off the breathlessness that may feel uncomfortable.

- *If you experience chronic pain, try exercise programs specifically for your needs.* You can find all kinds of excellent programs for exercise to help chronic pain, and many of them are completely free. First, get clearance from your doctor to begin, then check out some of the incredible resources you can find online. One of my favorites is *Yoga with Adriane* on YouTube (Mishler, n.d.). Adriane is down-to-earth, knowledgeable, and has videos for all types of chronic pain and other issues, including "Yoga for Headaches," "Yoga for Back Pain," and my favorite, "Yoga for a Bad Mood." And the best part? They're all free.

- *If you feel pain, ease up or stop.* If an exercise is painful, that's your body's way of saying, "Stop!" You may need to slow down, take a break, or rest for a day or two. You may also wish to switch to a lower-intensity exercise like walking, swimming, or water aerobics, which is very good for "good" and "bad" sore muscles. Remember: if pain persists, please seek medical advice from a doctor before resuming physical activity.

Sense of Self, Body Image, and Confidence

"I'm too self-conscious about how I look."
Many of us think that if we go to the gym everyone will be in super shape, and we'll feel like the odd man or woman out. We fear everyone will be watching us and commenting in their heads, or to each other, about our body or how we look. Let me bust this myth: it just isn't true. Most people at the gym are just like you. Most are not in super shape, and many are feeling the same way and thinking the same things as you. Hopefully, those at the gym are there to improve their own bodies and minds—not comment on others'.

Still, self-consciousness can be a major deterrent when it comes to exercise, and these suggestions can help:

- *Go solo.* Remember you don't have to workout in a gym or in public at all. If it's too uncomfortable, then avoid the crowds all together. Exercise at home with online videos, in your neighborhood, or invest in some home equipment like a treadmill, stationary bike, or elliptical machine. Check yard sales; people are always getting rid of exercise equipment because they don't use it, and you can benefit.
- *Focus on the future.* Imagine how you'll feel about yourself after you've been exercising for a while. Envision a healthy, happy, emotionally flourishing you, and give yourself credit for committing to this goal. Remember this vision when you feel uncomfortable and let it motivate you until your confidence eventually improves.
- *Review Key 2 and work through The Pyramid of Self-Worth.* Being aware that you're self-conscious is the first step in overcoming it. Practice self-acceptance and self-love using the tools in Key 3. As you grow in self-worth, you will grow in self-confidence.

"I feel insecure, stupid, etc . . .."
I think anyone who's ever been to a gym can relate to this one. You walk in and feel like everyone can tell you have no clue what you're

doing. You walk over to the machines and don't know how they work, or you look into an exercise class, but have no idea what the routine is. Even when I worked as a fitness instructor, I'd feel this when I went to a new gym. I always felt somewhat embarrassed, because I thought everyone could tell I had no idea what I was doing—yet.

As we keep repeating in this book, confidence is essential when it comes to exercise. We are much more motivated to exercise when we feel confident and secure in what we're doing. When we don't feel confident, the negative self-talk usually begins. Thoughts like, "I have no clue what I'm doing," "I am the worst one in this class, for sure," or "I look like an idiot!" can spiral us downward until our self-worth is completely dashed.

But, as we discussed at length in Key 5, we can choose to hear, challenge, and change unhealthy thoughts and self-talk. We can also remind ourselves that practice leads to increased confidence in exercise.

Here are some tips:

- *If you're too insecure for group exercise, then exercise alone or with a trusted friend.* I've heard of clients who were so insecure about how they looked when they exercised that they only tried it when they were completely alone. One client did push-ups in the bathroom so even his wife didn't see him as he tried to build up his confidence to go to the gym. Remember the story of Tyler, in Key 4? He started at home, too, and with practice, finally felt confident enough to go to the gym regularly. Remember, you don't have to go to a gym to get a good workout. (I don't use a gym at all these days.)
- *If you desire to go to the gym, then test it out in quiet times.* Take a tour so you can see where everything is and ask questions about how things work. Or, go when it's quiet and less busy at first, to give yourself time to get acquainted with things.
- *Remind yourself, "Practice makes better."* While practice may not make perfect, it certainly makes better, and exercise is no exception. The more you do each activity, the more comfortable you'll

become. Practice the exercises at home, if it's more comfortable, so you'll feel better prepared when you go to the gym. Over time, your confidence will build.

- *Tackle the negative self-talk.* Go back to Key 5 and review the tools for how to change your thoughts and beliefs. Use a thought record to keep track of your self-talk. Be honest, then review it and use "thought record, part two" to look for alternatives. If you're saying, "I am the worst one by far," then challenge it. You have no proof you're the worst, and what does it matter anyway? It's not a competition. You're only there to "beat" yourself (hopefully not to "beat" yourself up!). Instead, you might change it to, "I feel like I'm not good at this yet, but I know if I stick with it, I'll get better."

- *Try imagery or visualization.* Close your eyes, take a deep breath, and visualize yourself doing the activity you feel insecure about. Imagine the best-case scenario, where you know exactly what to do and you do it in a way that makes you feel confident and secure. Imagine yourself feeling confident about exercise in general as you practice and reach your exercise for mental health goals. Visit http://www.exercise4mentalhealth.com to download a podcast or watch a video of exercise for mental health visualizations.

"I'm afraid I'll fail."

Fear of failure, and sometimes even fear of success, is a powerful roadblock for many. Fear stops us in our tracks, no matter what its source. It falsely makes us believe we're protecting ourselves from some sort of harm, when the truth is fear only prevents potential good. Fear is not the same as a warning—that sense we get when something is truly wrong. When we feel a warning, we simply know something isn't right. Fear, however, is very chatty in our minds, reminding us of every reason we will never succeed.

Avoiding exercise because we're afraid we'll fail is the only failure when it comes to exercise for mental health. If we recognize that fear is only there to stop us from potentially achieving something great—in this case, mental health and happiness through exercise—then we can take back the control fear tries to exert over us and conquer the fear.

Even a fear of success can hold us back. Sometimes, we avoid exercise because we're afraid that if we succeed, we'll have to change, and change can be scary. But avoiding exercise because we're afraid of change is just another way of saying, "I guess I'll stay right where I am." It's the antithesis of progress, of improvement, of growth.

We must work to overcome fear if we want all the benefits exercise has to offer. Don't let fear get the best of you. Try these ideas and to help you face your fears:

- *Identify your fear.* "I'm afraid I'll be the laughing stock if I show up at the gym."
- *Name it for what it is.* Say, "This is fear, and fear only prevents good."
- *Feel the fear.* This can be tough at first, but sit still, breathe, and let the fear come into your body. Continue breathing as you FEEL the fear and remind yourself, "This is only an emotion. It's not me, and I won't let it control me." You may only be able to feel it for a moment before you push it away again, but keep coming back to it, little bits at a time, until you feel it loosen. As you process and feel the emotion, you take its power away. (For more on how to FEEL fear, see the steps above or watch "How to FEEL Powerful Emotions," at http://www.exercise4mentalhealth.com.)
- *Set realistic goals.* Sometimes, the reason we're afraid is because we've set our goals too high. Don't promise you're going to work-out hard everyday for an hour and then feel your self-worth plummet when you can't keep up. Go back and revisit Key 4 on goal-setting, and set goals that help reduce fear.

"I'm not athletic," or, "I'm just not an exerciser."

Many of us grow up believing we're just not made for exercise. Our body isn't as naturally agile or coordinated, or we just don't seem to get the same results as others. Identity labels such as "I'm not an athlete," "I'm not good at exercise," or "I just can't do it," are excuses that cut to the core of our self-worth, and furthermore, they're not true. We may not be as physically blessed as someone else, but we each have potential to gain the health and mental health benefits of exercise we desire, in our own unique way.

Here are some tips for coping with the urge to make excuses:

- *Use The Pyramid of Self-Worth to remind you who you really are.* Use the principles of self-awareness, self-acceptance, and self-love (Key 2) to remember that you are not the things you tell yourself. There is so much more to you, and you have the potential to exercise for life. Don't sell yourself short by giving up. Give yourself the benefit of the doubt that you are more than meets the eye. Then, practice self-awareness, self-acceptance, and self-love to overcome.

- *Keep it simple.* Start with basic activities, like walking, stretching, and lifting light weights, and take your time. Give your body time to adjust to what you're learning, and in time you will reach your goals.

- *Forget competition.* This isn't about competing with anyone, trying to be the superstar exerciser, or pumping so much iron you become the biggest guy at the gym. It's about the positive changes you work to create in your own body and mind—nothing else.

- *Find your unique strengths and build upon them to make exercise work for you.* Do activities that make you feel confident, comfortable, and happy about who you are. My mother-in-law is particularly good at pickleball, so she plays it every day, and usually wins. She may not be able to keep up with the hard bodies at the gym, but I'd like to see them try to keep up with her on the pickleball court. As you do activities you feel confident in, you'll begin to see you really are someone who exercises; it just may take a little experimenting to find your own way of doing it.

Social, Cultural, and Financial Concerns

"I don't have support."

You may experience people doubting you, tempting you away from exercise, or thanks to jealousy, hoping you'll fail. Perhaps exercise is not valued in your culture or family system, where even the ones you love most can't seem to support your choice to exercise for mental health. Ideally, you would be able to count on your spouse, partner, kids, family, and friends to support your choice to exercise, but if that's not the case, then perhaps these things can help:

- *Enlist any loved ones who are willing.* Explain your exercise for mental health goals and help loved ones understand how to help you. Ask them to check in and see how you're progressing. Encourage them to encourage you, or give you time and space for exercise. Or, invite them to exercise with you.
- *If your family and friends are not willing to be supportive, then seek support from others.* Seek out other friends, family members, coworkers, fitness professionals, and community groups where you can find support. The more varied and wide your support system, the better your chances for success.
- *Take a fitness class at a club, studio, or in your community where you can meet others who prioritize fitness.* Or, join a fitness-related club, like a skiing, running, or tennis club.
- *Find a "check-in" partner.* Select a trusted friend, coworker, or family member who also wants the benefits of exercise and set up a daily/weekly phone call to check in and report your exercise progress. Even if you exercise on your own, it can help to have someone to whom you are accountable.
- *Join an online exercise support group, like my "Exercise 4 Mental Health" Facebook group.* This is only one of many groups online where you can find support from others in the same situation. (To join my Facebook group, visit http://www.exercise4mental health.com and follow the link.)

"I can't afford a gym."

Hopefully by now you realize you don't have to have a gym membership to exercise. Here are some tips for alternative avenues for working out:

- *Use a home gym.* Above, we discussed how inexpensive it can be to set up a simple home gym. Many activities require no equipment at all, and most require only a few key pieces. You can even replace weights with inexpensive plastic tubing that can serve as resistance bands or use items you have at home, like full milk jugs. (In college, before I could afford weights, I lifted large shampoo bottles.)

- *Start an exercise group of your own.* Start a walking, swimming, or biking group, or form a class with friends. Several women I know started early morning exercise classes together with friends in their neighborhood. They set it up in someone's home and meet together three mornings a week to do aerobics and weight training.
- *Try a community center.* Classes offered at community facilities are often much more budget-friendly than private gyms, and often have just as much to offer.

Situational Roadblocks

"The weather is too awful to exercise."
Whether the weather is too hot, cold, humid, rainy, or snowy, there are plenty of good solutions to keep you moving:

- *Exercise indoors.* This is an obvious answer, because it's a good solution. If you need inspiration, try a YouTube exercise channel such as "Pop Sugar Fitness," (PopSugar Fitness, n.d.) which has all kinds of indoor exercise videos of different lengths and styles.
- *If you love the outdoors too much to give it up, then invest in weather-appropriate clothing.* Warm gear in the winter, rain gear in the spring, and cool gear in the summer can help you keep exercising—outdoors—all year long.
- *Pay attention to the time of day.* When it's hot in the summer, exercise first thing in the morning, and don't forget the sunscreen. In winter, midday is best, when it's warmest.

"I'm out of town all the time for work or travel, so I can't exercise."
Traveling can make it tricky, but it's no excuse not to exercise. In fact, lots of travel is hard on the body, and exercise can loosen you

up and help you de-stress. Here are some tips for making workouts happen on the road:

- *Pack resistance bands or a favorite DVD in your luggage.* These items require minimal space in a suitcase, and are lightweight. Workout in your hotel room.
- *Stay at hotels with a fitness room or pool.* Check ahead of time and then plan your exercise just like you would at home.
- *If you're flying, use layovers to take a brisk walk around the airport.* Your body will thank you, and your mind will feel refreshed.
- *Get out and explore.* I absolutely love getting out and walking around a new city. Sightseeing, visiting tourist attractions, or just taking in the local vibe on foot are all great ways to get your exercise in.

A Few Extra Ideas

Here are a few of the general things some of my Facebook followers suggested to make exercise more doable:

- "I want to get off medications. I remind myself of this everyday and it motivates me to exercise."
- "I remember that feeling of hitting 'rock bottom' and crying on the floor. I never want to be in that place again, so I exercise."
- "Paying for it helps. I'm more likely to go when I'm financially accountable."
- "I enjoy doing a fitness challenge—30, 60, 90 days. It has built-in support, and it becomes a game for me to not miss a day."
- "I tell myself to do the minimum viable workout and then to feel a sense of accomplishment for it. Even four minutes counts! Let yourself feel proud."
- "Put your workout clothes on right when you wake up, and wear running shoes during the day. You're much more likely to move!"
- "I have a playlist of music I love that I only let myself listen to when I'm working out. It's a fun way to reward myself for exercising."

- "I tell myself, 'Just 10 sit-ups.' Then, I sometimes stop, but more often I say, 'Okay, 10 more.'"
- "I join a walk, run, race, or even better, a team race, like a Ragnar race. Anything I need to prepare for motivates me. A mountain I'm working to climb."
- "Weigh-ins, photos, and accountability partners all help keep me motivated."
- "I tell myself, 'I'm doing this and I'm going to love it!'"
- "I reward myself with a good snack/energy food, and good music."
- "I remind myself that once I start, I always feel better."
- "I know I will feel less anxiety if I get out and do something active, and I remind myself."
- "I count housework as exercise. I make exercise into something that doesn't look like exercise."

When Exercise Becomes the Problem: Commitment versus Addiction

Sometimes, the roadblock is exercise itself. Over-exercising, or exercise addiction, is a serious problem that requires intervention in order to prevent injury or illness. There's a big difference between exercise commitment and exercise addiction.

Those who display exercise commitment consciously analyze the benefits of exercise, and develop a desire to receive such benefits. When a committed exerciser engages in an activity, she experiences satisfaction, achievement, and hopefully a little enjoyment as a result. All of these then motivate her to continue exercising (Szabo, 2000). Research explains that committed exercisers control their physical activity, often exercise for extrinsic rewards, see exercise as an important, but not central, part of their lives, and do not experience withdrawal symptoms when they stop (Szabo, 2000).

Conversely, exercise addiction involves behavior that is obsessive, compulsive, and causes significant impairment in one or more areas of life. Those with exercise addiction tend to: 1) exercise for internal satisfaction, though more as a drive or need than an experience of enjoyment; 2) see exercise as a main focus of life; 3) develop tolerance to the "feel good" chemicals of exercise; and 4) experience strong withdrawal symptoms when exercise is discontinued—like depression, anxiety, sleeplessness, tension, guilt, appetite loss, and headaches (Sachs, 1981). In short, those experiencing exercise addiction end up losing control over their physical activity behaviors (Sachs, 1981). Exercise addiction frequently co-occurs with eating disorders, another mental disorder focused on control, or lack thereof.

There are a number of hypotheses for why some become addicted to exercise. One is the endorphin hypothesis, which proposes that exercisers become addicted to the euphoric feelings produced by the increase of endorphins in exercise. In a sense, it views exercisers as "opiate junkies," and, similar to those addicted to drugs, the person begins to need more and more endorphins to experience the same (runner's) high. Another theory is called the sympathetic arousal hypothesis. This proposes that, because regular exercise leads to lower sympathetic arousal and a more relaxed resting state, over time, our bodies need more exercise to maintain an optimal level of arousal or to overcome lethargy at rest (Thompson & Blanton, 1987).

Whatever the cause, exercise addiction is something to watch out for. Use the "Exercise Addiction: What to Watch Out For" checklist, in the appendix of this book to help you determine if you're at risk. If you think you or someone you love may fit the criteria for over-exercising or exercise addiction, please seek help from a medical or mental health professional.

Exercise Success: It's All in Your Mind

The roadblocks above share a common core: they're all based on your thoughts, beliefs, and perceptions about exercise and your potential for success. As beneficial as exercise is *for* your mind, exercise success begins *with* your mind. When we open our eyes to this truth, we can begin to create a new mental structure that supports lasting motivation and dedication to exercise and mental health. No matter the challenge, with a little creativity, ingenuity, and work, it can be overcome.

Reflection Questions: Overcoming Roadblocks

1. What most prevents you from exercising? Are you short on time, energy, or motivation? Do you start a plan but always seem to give up? Do you hear negative thoughts creeping in, causing trouble? Identify all the roadblocks to your exercise success and list them in your journal, notebook, or below.

_____

_____

_____

_____

_____

_____

_____

_____

_____

_____

2. Brainstorm ideas for how you might overcome each roadblock, utilizing the suggestions presented above and including any personal ideas. No idea is too trivial. Include them all, and write them down.

_____

_____

_____

_____

_____

_____

3. Go back and select one roadblock to work on; then, select one or more ideas for how to overcome it. Do one thing right now to get you started. For example, if your biggest roadblock is motivation, you might call a friend and commit to go for a 20-minute bike ride tomorrow. Make it firm, and implement a reasonable consequence for yourself if you don't do what you've said you would. Start slowly, but start today.

PART 3

Exercise for Life

KEY 7

GET FITT—PHYSICALLY
AND MENTALLY

"Exercise to stimulate, not to annihilate. The world wasn't formed in a day, and neither were we. Set small goals and build upon them."

—Lee Haney

Finally! We're ready to create an exercise program that works for you. Why did I wait to introduce the fundamentals of creating an exercise routine until Key 7? Remember the Transtheoretical Model of Change we discussed in Key 5? That's why. Because "action" isn't stage one. It's stage four, and if we want lasting change, we must take action only after the stages of "Precontemplation," "Contemplation," and "Preparation."

As we've worked through the first six keys to mental health through exercise, we've also been moving through the stages of the Transtheoretical Model of Change. Or, at least, these keys have provided us with the information and tools that can get us started moving through the spiral of change—if we desire. Similar to a key ring, it's up to us to find the right keys, insert, and turn them, in order to unlock the doors we want to enter. In this case, all eight keys work together to unlock the doors to long-term exercise and robust mental health.

We first had to understand, in Part 1. In Key 1, we learned the facts on what exercise can do for our mental health—how it improves our body, mind and spirit. This opened the door from precontemplation to contemplation. We were then able to contemplate how physical activity has impacted our sense of self-worth, and vice versa (Key 2), and how our exercise and mental health values and attitudes have been impacted by, or have impacted, our family relationships (Key 3). Part 2 provided the keys to help us prepare for exercise—by learning and practicing the necessary skills to build motivation, set specific, achievable goals, change faulty beliefs, and overcome the roadblocks that stand in our way (Keys 4 through 6).

Now, we're ready to finish our preparation by creating an exercise plan to fit each of our unique circumstances and needs, using The FITT principle. We'll learn more about the FITT principle below, but in general, FITT outlines the elements of a well-balanced, effective exercise plan. It can help us use the goal-setting skills we began developing in Key 4 to create a specific, achievable exercise for mental health plan that works for you.

First, let's take a look at the recommended guidelines for physical activity to give us an idea of what your exercise plan might entail. Once again, I want to remind you to please seek your doctor's approval before beginning any new exercise program or significantly changing your existing exercise routine. I've said it before, and I'm saying again, because it's that important. Seek counsel from your doctor on how to best apply the information in this key to keep you safe, prevent injury or illness, and help you reach your optimal exercise for mental health potential.

Exercise Recommendations

The Center for Disease Control (CDC, 2011) provides exercise recommendations, which are a helpful place to begin when setting up an exercise plan. These guidelines are here to do just that—serve as a guide. They are here to show you what is generally recommended for optimal exercise benefits. They are not here to make you feel badly about yourself, feel like you're not doing enough, or overwhelm you. They are here to show you what the general population should be striving for. If, for any reason, you're not ready to exercise according to these recommendations, it's okay. They can be something to shoot for, a starting place, or a building place; it all depends on your current exercise and mental health situation.

One thing I appreciate about the CDC recommendations is that they offer different options for total exercise time, intensity, type, and frequency, so you can customize them to work for you. Focus on the option(s) you believe are best suited to you, and stick with me as we explore the FITT principle. It will help us better understand these guidelines and how to apply them, specifically, to create your exercise for mental health plan.

Generally, for adults, exercise should consist of:

- *Moderate-intensity aerobic exercise,* such as fast walking or cycling: two hours and 30 minutes (or 150 minutes) every week.
- *Strength-training exercises,* such as lifting weights, push-ups, or using resistance bands: two or more days each week, working all the major muscle groups.

OR you may choose to do:

- *High-intensity aerobic exercise,* such running, jogging, or swimming laps: one hour and 15minutes (75 minutes) a week, along with the recommended two or more days of strength-training exercises

OR you may choose to do:

- A mix of the two options above.

For even greater physical and mental health benefits, and if cleared by your doctor, you may opt to:

- *Increase your cardiovascular activity,* per week, to either: 300 minutes of moderate-intensity activity plus two or more days of strength training, or 150 minutes of high-intensity cardio plus strength training, or a mix of these two options.

(For childhood and elderly adult exercise recommendations, see appendix.)

These recommendations focus on making exercise part of a weekly routine and not just a daily one, which implies that if you skip a day (or two, or three), it doesn't mean you've failed. You still have the rest of the week to meet your exercise for mental health goal. The most important thing when it comes to exercise for adults is to avoid inactivity, according to the Office of Disease Prevention and Health Promotion (ODPHP) (2008). As we've discussed in previous chapters, exercise consists of anything that gets us up and moving. Total exercise time can, and should, include: work-related movement—taking the stairs or doing a walking meeting; family-related movement—playing tag with your kids or going for a family swim; home-related movement—vigorous house-cleaning or gardening; and social movement—going for a hike with friends.

The FITT Principle is a helpful tool in making sure we meet these recommendations, and in creating an exercise for mental health plan.

Get FITT

The FITT Principle is the underlying foundation of exercise, the "rules" by which exercise is governed and the key to exercise programs that work. FITT stands for: Frequency, Intensity, Time, and Type. The CDC guidelines, above, incorporate each of the FITT elements, and understanding these four components enables us to mold them into the perfect recipe for individual exercise for mental health success.

Let's take a look at each component of the FITT principle:

Frequency

In general, three to five days a week is recommended for cardiovascular, or aerobic, exercise. Your exercise frequency will depend, of course, on your fitness level and mental health needs and goals.

When you're beginning an exercise for mental health program, three days a week is a good place to start, but as I've said throughout this book, the most important thing when it comes to exercise frequency is to move as often as you can. Exercising only two days a week is still better than nothing, and soon, you might increase to three days, and then perhaps, four or five. Many people exercise moderately at least six days a week, leaving one day off, while some exercise every single day, because it makes them feel so much better. It's all up to you.

Strength training is also recommended, two to three times a week, with at least 48 hours in between sessions to let your muscles recover. But again, this is something to work up to if you're just getting started. (More on cardiovascular and strength training exercises, below.)

Intensity

Short answer: you should exercise just outside of your comfort level. I say "just outside," because if you stay completely comfortable, then you're probably not pushing yourself quite enough to really get the most from exercise.

Of course, "comfort level" is completely relative. For some, just outside your "comfort level" means walking slowly up the driveway and back, and that is perfectly fine when you're just beginning. The goal is to first, push yourself to move, and then, when you're ready, push yourself to move just a tad more intensely, building your exercise strength and stamina, and reaping greater and greater mental health benefits as you go.

Ideally, you will exercise in your target heart rate zone, which is based on your age and fitness level. Another way to measure heart rate, or intensity, is the rate of perceived exertion (RPE) scale.

When exercising, ask yourself, "How do I feel right now?" and rate it on a scale, from 1 through 10. For optimum fitness and mental health results, cardiovascular exercise should be performed at a 7 to 9 on the RPE scale. A 7 would be, "I can talk while I'm exercising, but it's pretty uncomfortable to do so," whereas a 9 would be, "I can barely talk at all." A 10 is fine for short bursts of intensity, as in interval training, but will wear you out quickly and can be harmful for extended periods of time. Especially when first beginning, it's important to check in regularly and make sure you keep the intensity of your exercise at a manageable level.

Rate of Perceived Exertion Chart

10	Very, Very Strenuous Activity Completely out of breath, Unable to talk
9	Very Strenuous Activity Able to speak only one word at a time Very out of breath
7-8	Strenuous Activity Can speak a sentence or two at a time Breathing heavily
4-6	Moderate Activity Can talk and carry on a conversation Breathing rate increased, but not heavy
2-3	Light Activity Easy breathing Can talk and converse easily
1	No Activity

Christina G. Hibbert, Psy.D., 2015

When it comes to strength training, intensity refers to: 1) the amount of weight you lift, 2) how many different types of exercises you do, and 3) the number of repetitions, or sets, for each exercise. Again, this will vary greatly, depending on your current exercise and mental health needs and goals. In general, starting with one or two sets of each exercise, working all the major muscle groups each week by doing multiple types of exercises (i.e. biceps, triceps, back, chest, legs, and so on), is ideal. As we'll discuss below, the number of reps and sets you do, as well as how heavy the weights you use, impact the intensity of the exercise. If you're new to strength training start slowly and seek help from a trainer, instructor, or friend to ensure you do the exercises correctly. Don't overdo it at first. Over time, you can build your strength training intensity, if you like. (More on strength training below.)

Time

When it comes to receiving the mental health benefits of exercise, 30 minutes of moderate intensity exercise, three days a week, can do the trick. That's only 90 minutes a week. The best part is that these blocks don't have to be continuous; three 10-minute blocks of activity can be just as effective as one 30-minute block (Sharma et al., 2006).

It also helps to look at total exercise time per week, as opposed to daily exercise time. Some days, you might exercise for only 15 minutes, while other days, you'll get in an hour. Even the CDC recommendations, above, use a weekly total when it comes to exercise time, so remember you can be flexible as long as you make up for it.

It helps to break exercise into aerobic and anaerobic time when you're looking to do more than the minimum required to receive the mental health payoffs. When doing aerobic, or cardiovascular exercise, it's suggested that you work at a high enough intensity to increase your heart rate and keep it up for 20 minutes or more (use the RPE chart to monitor your heart rate intensity). Twenty to 50 minutes of sustained cardiovascular exercise per session is ideal, with a five-minute warm up before and at least a five-minute cool down and stretch after.

Again, research shows that this can be broken up into 10-minute blocks and be just as effective—twice a day for high-intensity cardio, such as running, or three times a day for moderate-intensity cardio, such as walking (Garber et al., 2011). One intriguing study showed that even 10 minutes of easy aerobic exercise with only one minute of intense cardio, three times per week, improved overall health in overweight adults (Gillen et al., 2014). Once again, the most important thing is to move—even for a few minutes at a time. It all adds up, and what it adds up to is greater mental and physical health.

For anaerobic or strength training exercise, like weight lifting, time will vary according to the muscle groups worked. A workout focused on one or two muscle groups at a time, such as legs and back, may only take 15 to 20 minutes; whereas, a workout for the entire body may take an hour. It's okay, and even suggested, to vary the time and find what works best for you.

Type

If it isn't clear by now, then let me say it one more time: do whatever type of exercise you'll do. Whatever you enjoy, holds your interest, keeps you moving—do *that*. The best exercise programs contain three main types of exercise each week: aerobic (or cardiovascular) exercise, anaerobic exercise (or strength training), and flexibility training. Variety is important not only to keep us interested and motivated to exercise, but also to keep our muscles and minds working, enabling us to get the greatest physical and mental health benefits from exercise.

Aerobic, or cardiovascular, exercise increases our heart rate for a sustained period of time. Cardiovascular exercise is crucial for a healthy heart and mind. Walking is considered a great cardio exercise to begin with; it's easy on the joints and you can take it at your

own pace. Even Thomas Jefferson said, "Walking is the best possible exercise. Habituate yourself to walk very far" (Thomas Jefferson's Monticello, n.d.).

But walking isn't the only cardio exercise. Different types of
cardio include: swimming, jogging, running, dancing, aerobics
classes, water aerobics, Zumba, basketball, soccer, tennis, elliptical
trainers, hiking, biking, rowing, interval training—the list goes on.
Even Pilates and power yoga can be aerobic, if you keep moving
and work at a high enough level of intensity.

Anaerobic exercise, or strength training, increases muscle mass
and physical strength. It also relieves tension and stress in the body,
which benefits us mentally and physically (Thayer, 2001). Strength
training uses weights, resistance bands, or body weight to increase
bone mass and strengthen muscles. Examples of strength training
exercises include: push-ups, pull-ups, chair dips, squats, lunges,
calf raises, sit-ups, crunches, core training, resistance band work,
and weight lifting. It's important to work all major muscle groups
when doing anaerobic exercise, including the shoulders, arms
(biceps and triceps), back, abdomen, buttocks, and legs (ham-
strings, quads, and calves), and let your muscles rest for at least 48
hours in between workouts so you don't get overly sore or injured.

Strength training also uses sets and repetitions, or reps. Reps
refer to how many times you do a specific exercise; for instance, 10
bicep curls is 10 reps. Sets refers to how many times you do each
group of reps; for example, three sets of 10 reps means you'll do 10
curls, three times, with breaks in between. The amount of sets you
do will depend on your exercise goals, but even one full set of each
muscle group can bring improvement and mental health benefits.
Those wishing to add muscle mass should use heavier weights and
do 8 to 10 reps per set. For leaner muscle tone, 12 to 15 reps with
lighter weights is recommended.

And remember, strength training is for men and women.
Though often associated more with men, strength training is particularly helpful for women, allowing us to stay trim and fit by
strengthening core muscles and bones, helping prevent osteoporo-

sis, and decreasing stress and tension in the body and mind. So, ladies, if you've never tried it before, it's something you should definitely consider.

Flexibility training, or stretching, is usually the most neglected of the three main types of exercise. We feel we don't have time, or perhaps don't recognize the importance of flexibility training to our overall mental and physical health. Regular stretching keeps our muscles lean and limber. It improves range of motion and prevents those short, penguin-like steps we see older people taking when they've lost the flexibility to walk in strides. Stretching prevents injury, improves chronic pain, and helps us relax. Flexibility exercises like yoga, Pilates, dance, and light stretching are not only good for elongating all muscle groups and preventing injury; they can decrease anxiety, stress, and worry, increase mental clarity, calmness, and energy, and promote overall wellness and happiness.

It is recommended to stretch daily, or at least several times a week, and to always stretch after exercise. Before exercise it's more important to do light cardio to get your muscles warmed up, but after the workout, when your muscles are nice and warm, is the perfect time to stretch. Never stretch cold muscles, for it can lead to injury. To incorporate more flexibility exercise into your week: warm up first thing in the morning and stretch; take stretch breaks throughout the day; sit in front of your favorite television show and stretch in the evening; or stretch lightly just before bed.

One final type of exercise is balance exercises, like Tai Chi or yoga poses. These are also important to consider, especially as we get older (Harvard Health Publications, 2015), for they keep our minds and bodies fresh and focused. Including balance exercises in your weekly routine is a great way to keep your mind sharp and promote overall balance in your life.

Applying the FITT Principle

In the same way that the eight keys to mental health through exercise contribute to and build upon one another, the components of

FITT are also dependent upon each another, and can work together to help you create an effective exercise plan. As you can see, the FITT principle provides not only guidance for creating an exercise program—it provides options. The trick is to use these options to create the best plan for your unique exercise for mental health goals.

When using the FITT principle, it's important to understand the following:

- *Each of the FITT components—frequency, intensity, time, and type—influences and is influenced by one another.* In other words, the type of exercise I do will impact the intensity, time, and frequency; the intensity of the exercise I do will impact the time, frequency, and type, and so on. If I go walking on a flat street, it will be less intense than walking up a steep hill. I'm still walking, but the intensity increases based on my circumstances. I will still feel the mental health benefits of walking, either way, but if I want greater benefits I'll need to walk longer, more intensely, or more frequently on the flat surface to get the same benefits I'll receive from walking up a steep hill, in less time.
- *The total weekly amount of exercise counts most when it comes to physical and mental health with FITT.* More than the frequency, intensity, or type of exercise, total weekly fitness time (including aerobic, strength training, flexibility, and balance) is most important when it comes to receiving the physical and mental health benefits exercise provides (ODPHP, 2008).
- *There are countless ways to set up a weekly exercise routine using FITT.* When beginning, you may choose to do cardiovascular exercise three days a week, for two, 10-minute blocks, and then to do push-ups and sit-ups twice a week for 10 minutes. You may wish to focus on strength training and do all the muscle groups, three days a week, with shorter cardio sessions on two days. Or, you may do cardio and strength training on the same day, three days a week, stretching or doing yoga two other days. The possibilities are endless.
- *Choose activities that you enjoy.* I know I keep saying this over

and over, but it's important. As we have seen, there are a multitude of options when it comes to exercise, and you're more likely to stick with exercise for mental health when you do activities you enjoy. Seek to include some cardio, strength, and flexibility exercises each week. If you're not sure what you enjoy, then start investigating.

- *Start with small time segments—even a few minutes at a time— and build from there.* Move at your own pace, and track exercise time over the whole week rather than one day. Get up, reduce sedentary behaviors, and increase movement. Eventually, if you add a little at a time, you'll be exercising regularly most days every week.

- *Start with lower intensity workouts and work your way up.* You don't have to start by running three miles or doing heavy weight lifting. In fact, you shouldn't. The RPE scale is a great tool for making sure you're not overdoing it. Shoot for a "4-6," to start. As you get more accustomed to exercise, work your way up to a "7-8." As your body adjusts to the physical activity, you'll find that the exertion you feel will also adjust, and activities that once felt like a 9 will begin to feel like a 6. This is why this chart is so helpful—it changes and grows along with you.

Ponder This . . . The FITT Principle

Ask yourself, "How might the FITT principle help me set up an effective, doable exercise plan?"

Other Important Elements of Creating an Exercise Program

Creating your exercise for mental health plan will involve the FITT principle, but there are several other important things to know about exercise before you jump in:

Warm Up and Cool Down

Many people skip this part of exercise, but it's essential to a healthy exercise routine. Warm up by walking, jogging in place, or doing jumping jacks for five minutes. Then, your muscles will be pliable and ready for whatever you're ready to bring. After your workout, spend at least five minutes stretching all the muscle groups you worked. Stretching is critical in preventing injury and soreness, and it's also part of a balanced exercise plan.

Invest in Comfortable, Well-Fitting Shoes

When I used to teach aerobics, we were encouraged to buy new exercise shoes every six months. Now that I'm on a more "normal" exercise routine, I replace them about once every year. Proper footwear prevents injury and increases comfort, and shoes can wear out faster than most of us realize. You may also consider wearing workout shoes on weekends or when you're at home. My good friend, Becky, says that she wears her running shoes as much as possible when she's at home. "If I have them on, I'm more likely to run to the mailbox or run up and down the stairs, getting more exercise in," she says.

Wear Comfortable Clothing
That is Weather-Appropriate, and Layer

Make yourself comfortable by wearing ideal clothing. In warmer weather, make sure your clothing is not too tight or hot. In cooler weather, wear layers so you can adjust as your body temperature rises. For safety reasons, wear bright, reflective clothing in the early morning or when exercising at night.

Music is Motivation

For many people, music is what gets them going. Putting on your favorite tunes is a great way to get you pumped and ready to go.

Also, after a while, your body will be conditioned to want to work out to those specific songs—a win-win. If music isn't your thing, then you might like exercising to audiobooks or podcasts.

Incorporate Meditation and Stillness

Not everyone wants to exercise to music. For some, exercise is a quiet, spiritual connection or inspiration time. I get my best ideas when I'm outside going for a walk or jog, so use exercise wisely when you need a little more peace or insight.

You Don't Have to Exercise at a Gym or Hire a Personal Trainer

Exercising at a gym or with a personal trainer are great options for many people, motivating and pushing them in ways they couldn't do alone. But it's not an option, or a desire, for everyone, and it's definitely not necessary. Exercise at home, using DVDs or You-Tube videos, get outdoors and obtain the benefits of sunlight therapy, join a team sport, or just work out wherever suits you best and keeps you doing it.

If You Want Continued Improvement, Vary the FITT Components Using the "5% More" Rule

Once the FITT elements are all in play you will see improvement as your body adapts to your exercise plan, and this is our goal. However, if you want to continue to see improvement, you have to change one or more elements of FITT. Our muscles and mind get used to the activity we provide, and our improvement can, and will, eventually plateau. One rule of thumb I like to use is "5% more." Increase any element of FITT by just 5% at a time, and over time, you'll continue to improve in physical and mental health.

Mix it up by incorporating a new type of exercise and rotating (i.e. jogging one day, weight training the next, and then yoga).

Varying the types of workouts and exercises you do each week keeps your mind and body guessing and you interested. You may also add more frequent sessions of exercise, increase total exercise time, or try higher intensity workouts.

If You've Reached Your Fitness Goals and Like Where You Are, Then Stick With the Same Exercise Program

I know many people who've done the exact same exercise plan for years, and it works. In fact, when it comes to mental health, many people stick with the same exercise program as part of their must-do everyday routine. They know all too well that if they stop their program, the benefits to their mental health will fade away, too.

FITT Strategies for Specific Mental Health Concerns

Some mental illnesses or challenges respond better to a certain exercise type, time, frequency, or intensity. The FITT principle can, and should, be tailored for your specific mental health needs. Knowing these can help you find the FITT that is right for you.

Depression

- Higher intensity, longer workouts seem most effective in treating depression. Running and walking are the exercises most highly correlated with decreased depression, but studies show that any type of aerobic and/or anaerobic exercise helps (Leith, 2009).
- Even 20 minutes of brisk walking, three days a week, has been shown to improve overall psychological health and decrease depression (Craft & Perna, 2004).
- If you're experiencing increased stress, moodiness, or depression and feel you're no longer getting the benefits you once were, you may be overtraining. It's good to shorten and vary

your workouts to keep your body and mind from plateauing (Olderman, 2014).

Anxiety

- Those with anxiety should avoid high intensity workouts, at least at first. It may trigger anxiety symptoms in some (Otto & Smitts, 2011).
- Participating consistently in a variety of mild to moderate aerobic exercises over time, however, has been shown to significantly reduce one's sensitivity to anxiety, so stay with it (Otto & Smitts, 2011; Leith, 2009).
- Exercises like yoga, Pilates, stretching, and lifting weights are helpful to calm anxiety, teach relaxation skills, and reduce body and muscle tension.

Schizophrenia and Personality Disorders

- When it comes to schizophrenia and personality disorders, jogging is associated with greatest improvements. Aerobic exercise, in general, seems most effective in this population, as it appears to increase a sense of self-efficacy and self-sufficiency (Leith, 2012).
- Research shows that a longer-term exercise plan is more effective with schizophrenia because it improves energy, increases fitness, and helps combat obesity, which can be a problem in those taking antipsychotic medications. In one study, schizophrenic patients who completed a three-month exercise program showed improved fitness levels, exercise tolerance, and increased energy levels overall (Fogarty et al., 2004).

Bipolar Disorders

- Bipolar disorder, types I and II, can especially benefit from exercise—by increasing self-esteem, improving fitness, and providing much needed mood-boosting endorphins and neurotransmitters.

- Make sure to talk with your doctor before you begin, and if you're on a medication like lithium, be sure to stay hydrated.
- Don't make it complicated; just make it part of your daily "musts." Even a simple walk around the block once or twice a day can make a huge impact, if done consistently (Krans, 2012).

Grief

- High intensity workouts are especially helpful for those suffering from grief. They can get you into the sun and around other people, get you out of your foggy, dark, isolated head, and remind you that you're strong and will be well (Mercola, 2014).
- The added benefits of endorphins and increased serotonin in the brain are also helpful in treating grief.

Substance Abuse

- Cardio, yoga, and outdoor exercises are especially recommended for those overcoming substance abuse disorders. Vigorous cardio relieves stress, strengthens the heart, keeps weight down, and helps toxic chemicals sweat out of the body (Recovery Ranch, 2015).
- Yoga is a calming exercise, and getting outside helps calm and energize the body and mind (Recovery Ranch, 2015).

Eating Disorders

- When beginning a program for eating disorders treatment, it's important to involve your medical or mental health provider, who can teach you how to keep exercise from becoming too strenuous, unhealthy, or intense.
- Walking is the most recommended exercise for eating disordered individuals, because it is calming and has less potential for abuse. Also, yoga, Pilates, stretching and low-impact aerobics are good options for dealing with underlying anxiety and teaching a healthy mind-body connection (Rader Programs, 2015).

Create your Exercise for Mental Health Plan

Now, we're finally ready to use everything we've learned so far to create your "Exercise for Mental Health Plan." We will pull from all the keys and activities in this book, so first, gather all the activities you've completed from Keys 1 through 6. Then, use the "Exercise 4 Mental Health Plan" worksheet provided below, or download one from http://www.exercise4mentalhealth.com. Work through the following steps, using your worksheet or notebook:

1. *Identify your mental health goals.* Revisit the mental health goals you wrote down in Key 4 and apply them here. These will help you determine which FITT components will work best for you. Write them on your worksheet.

2. *Review your exercise goals.* Revisit Key 4 and the exercise goals you wrote down. This includes your desires for physical and mental well-being as they relate to exercise. Do you desire to start running for the first time ever, because you believe it will keep your mind more stable and focused? Are you looking to reduce worry and tension in your body by lifting weights? Or are you just looking to do the bare minimum each week to help you reach your mental health goals? Whatever your exercise goals, make them clear, specific, and make sure they're achievable.

3. *Using the mental health and the exercise goals you've already set forth, use FITT to create specific exercise for mental health goals.* For instance, if your main mental health goal is to overcome the grief of your divorce, and your main exercise goal is to start swimming, then you might start by setting a goal to swim for 20 minutes, three days a week, doing whatever stroke is "doable" for you to keep it up. Eventually, you might work up to swimming the breaststroke, freestyle, and then butterfly stroke in 10-minute increments, for 30 minutes total. If your primary mental health goal is to experience more calm and mental clarity, then you may opt for doing yoga three days a week and walking two days, instead.

4. *Write specific exercise for mental health goals, using FITT.* Use

the following sentence to make sure your goals are specific and incorporate all the elements of FITT: "I will do _____ (type of exercise), at _____ level (easy, moderate, difficult intensity), for _____ minutes (time), _____ times a week (frequency)."

5. *Identify and prepare for potential roadblocks.* What roadblocks do you anticipate? What strategies will you employ to overcome challenges? Use the activities from Key 6 to help you identify the problems that may come your way, and then prepare by writing down strategies you plan to use in response.

6. *Build mental fortitude and motivation.* As we discussed in Keys 4 through 6, exercise is just as much a mental activity as it is physical. That's why we worked so hard to build motivation and thought-changing skills. Now, it's time to employ these skills. Sometimes, the only thing that gets us up and moving is a single thought in our mind, telling us we can do it. What thoughts or truthful affirmations will you use to foster your exercise success? Revisit Key 5 and your list of truthful affirmations, and add those that feel most helpful to your exercise plan. When your body feels unmotivated, pull out your affirmations and let your mind talk your body into exercise.

7. *Sometimes, you have to move your body in order to move your mind.* It works both ways. If we can motivate our mind, we're more likely to move our body, but sometimes, we have to move our body in order to move our mind. Sometimes the simple act of standing up and walking to the door frees our mind of the paralyzing thoughts that we "can't do it." Sometimes, it's putting on our running shoes. Sometimes, it's stretching on the floor. When your mind feels stuck, use your body to get free.

8. *Set a deadline, and be accountable.* When will you check in on your progress—how often, and with whom? Set a specific deadline for each goal, and make yourself accountable to someone else, if possible. You may set your own goals and tell your spouse about them, or you may set goals with a friend or a group you exercise with.

9. *Reward yourself once you achieve a goal.* Don't skip this impor-

tant step. You've worked hard, and you deserve a reward once you've achieved a goal. Do something that is meaningful to you, treat yourself to something you love, or go and celebrate with a friend or loved one. Take time to reflect and really soak in all that you have achieved, and have received, as a result.

My Exercise for Mental Health Plan

Date: _____

My top three mental health goals are: (i.e. to feel less depressed, reduce anxiety, increase energy or clarity, keep myself stable, increase happiness, and so on)

_____
_____
_____
_____
_____
_____
_____
_____
_____
_____
_____
_____
_____

To help me achieve these mental health goals, I plan to exercise by: (i.e. walking every day, doing yoga three times a week, lifting weights twice a week, and so on)

_____
_____
_____
_____

_____
_____
_____
_____
_____
_____
_____
_____
_____
_____

Write each exercise goal, above, into a statement like the following: "I will do _____ (type of exercise), at _____ intensity level (low, moderate, high), for _____ minutes (time), _____ times a week (frequency)."

_____
_____
_____
_____
_____
_____
_____
_____
_____
_____
_____
_____
_____

Potential roadblocks I see for these goals include:

_____
_____
_____
_____

_____

_____

_____

_____

I will seek to overcome these roadblocks by:

_____

_____

_____

_____

_____

_____

_____

_____

_____

The following strategies, affirmations, and beliefs will help me stick with my goals:

_____

_____

_____

_____

_____

_____

_____

_____

_____

I will achieve the goals on this plan by _____
_____ (deadline/date), and I will be accountable to _____
(accountability partner) by _____

_____

_____

_____ (what you will do to check in—i.e. call, text, talk once a week, or once a month, etc.).

Once I reach each goal, I will reward myself by:

_____

_____

_____

_____

_____

_____

_____

I will follow this plan, continually evaluate, and make necessary changes until I achieve my exercise for mental health goals.

Signed: _____

Case Examples

If there's nothing else you gain from this book, I hope you at least come to fully comprehend that every one of us is unique. We each have our own needs, struggles, goals, and paths to reaching those goals. As I share a few stories from those who have reached their exercise for mental health goals, you will see how each and every exercise for mental health plan will look and feel different, and how that's exactly as it should be.

"Listen to Your Body"—Lindsay's Story

Lindsay was half way through her third pregnancy when she delivered her stillborn child. Prior to this tragedy, she had been a yoga instructor and loved the calm, centered way she felt after yoga. But for the first time in her life, Lindsay no longer wanted to hear her thoughts during exercise. Friends suggested kickboxing, so she could pound out her grief, and it helped. "Having a community and friends in the class helped me channel my sorrow into strength and kick butt," she says. "Interestingly, however, I realized that I no longer had that mind-body connection I used to have, and desperately needed. Kickboxing, for me, was just a mindless way to get the grief out."

Eventually, Lindsay was able to get pregnant again, but the road to rediscovering the mind-body connection with exercise was long and winding. She started working out with a trainer and lifting weights, and loved the slow, deliberate movements. They reminded her of yoga and re-formed that mind-body link for her. She started with light weights, and then heavier weights and all was going well, until her trainer started adding in more cardiovascular exercises. "I hated it," Lindsay says. "I tried all kinds of cardio, but the more I did, the more my brain would scream at me to stop! I just wanted to lift heavy weights." Lindsay says she felt physically sick when she'd increase her cardio workouts, and eventually was on the brink of quitting altogether.

Luckily, she worked with her trainer to find a solution for her specific needs. Lindsay focused more of her time on weight lifting and then started rollerblading around her neighborhood, listening to music. "I only do it for 15 to 20 minutes, but I like getting outside and seeing friends and nature while I get some cardio," Lindsay says. Part of Lindsay's exercise for mental health plan also includes nutrition. "I was diagnosed with Celiac disease a couple years ago," Lindsay says, "so I'm motivated to focus on nutrition, and that has made a huge difference." As she's focused on nutrition and exercise, her body and mind have felt connected once more. "Your body will tell you what it needs if you listen," Lindsay says. "My body has needed different types of workouts at different stages of my life, and when I listen to my body, it all works out."

"Gradually Add On"—Terry's Story

Terry had been struggling with severe PTSD for months when he tried exercising for the first time. Previously, Terry had been only mildly active, but since his PTSD diagnosis, even the smallest increase in his heart rate sent him into a full-blown panic attack. Getting to the gym was not even a question—it was way too scary to not only face his exercise fears, but do so in public. But he knew he needed to move and build strength if he was ever going to get some control back in his life.

So, he started at home, with free weights and floor exercises. At first he could only do 10 reps of each exercise—biceps, triceps, and back—three days a week. Over a few months, he built up to three sets of 10 reps of a dozen exercises, three to five days a week. As his physical strength improved, he felt more emotionally contained and was able to start walking. It was a challenge, but he started small, allowing himself to saunter around the block and quit if he felt panic coming on. Gradually, he increased the distance and the pace until he was walking a couple of brisk miles, three days a week, and lifting weights for 45 minutes, three days a week.

"Progress, Not Perfection"—Barb's Story

Barb is close a friend of mine who was diagnosed with a serious heart condition in her late twenties. She was overweight, in poor physical health, and feeling down about herself. Barb was also in heavy grief, since she'd been told she shouldn't have any more children. Barb did not enjoy exercise and especially detested running, but learning that she could literally die if she didn't do something to improve her health gave her the motivation to begin.

Barb started by walking three days a week, for 20 minutes, "and it was miserable," she says. Her heart condition made it hard for her to breathe, and any physical activity only seemed to make it worse. "But I kept at it, because even though I was grief-stricken from learning I couldn't have any more children, and even though I literally struggled to breathe, I knew that exercise was the only way I could live long enough to raise the children I already had. I told myself, 'Get up and walk. You'll feel happier and enjoy your kids more today if you do.'"

And she did. Barb posted the motto, "Strive for progress, not perfection," on her fridge, and worked her way up to walking longer and farther most days of the week, even when she didn't feel like it. Eventually, she tried jogging and was surprised to find that, even though she still struggled for breath, when she was done, she felt even better. She was able to work through her grief by literally strengthening her heart.

Today, Barb is an avid runner. She's even started swimming, to train for an Iron Woman competition. Her heart is physically healthy, and emotionally, her heart has healed, too. "Before, my mind gave up way before my body did. I used to think, 'I can't do it' and, I believed myself. Now, I've proven that's not true. Over time, and with a lot of small steps, I've proven that my body can do far more than I ever dreamed." She's in the best physical shape of her life, her heart is doing wonderfully, her self-confidence is through the roof, and even on those days when grief or heartache creep back in, Barb knows she can push through, and so she does.

Exercise for Life

The bottom line is: whatever you'll actually do, whenever you'll actually do it, that is where you begin. Then, you vary the type, add a little more time, intensity, or frequency, and before you know it, you're seeing progress, or rather, feeling it.

As Benjamin Franklin said, "Energy and persistence conquer all things" (Goodreads, 2015). Never give up. There's always a way, if you keep on looking. That's what Key 8 is all about—remaining dedicated to exercise for mental health your whole life long.

Reflection Questions: Creating your Plan

1. Review the "Exercise for Mental Health Plan" you set up. Do you feel like it's missing anything? Does it seem achievable? Specific? Do you need to add or change anything? Do you believe the plan can work? Why or why not?

   _____

   _____

   _____

_____

_____

_____

_____

_____

_____

_____

_____

_____

2. What are your biggest strengths when it comes to creating an exercise plan that works? How can you best use these strengths?

_____

_____

_____

3. What are your biggest weaknesses? How can you best overcome them?

_____

_____

_____

_____

_____

_____

KEY 8

IMPLEMENT YOUR
VISION AND FLOURISH

"Continuous effort—not strength or intelligence—is the key to unlocking our potential."

—Winston Churchill

This is it—the last key to mental health through exercise, and it's all about implementing your plan, maintaining it, and flourishing in exercise and mental health your whole life long.

We've been inspired by the many benefits of exercise for mental health; we've learned to challenge and overcome mental and physical roadblocks. We've learned to retrain our brains and how we think about exercise, influencing how we feel and what we do about exercise, and we've learned how to create an exercise program that keeps us FITT for life.

Now, we look to the future. We look to stages four and five of the Transtheoretical Model of Change—to action and maintenance. Once you've taken action and implemented your plan, it's time to ensure you'll maintain it. If you have yet to take action on your exercise for mental health plan, there's no time like the present. But, how do we stay dedicated to exercise for mental health, long-term? It's one of the biggest questions for many of us.

The Power of Dedication

Dedication is the power we have to stick with exercise even when we don't feel like it, our mental health isn't in ideal shape, and life challenges arise. For many people, dedication is a huge barrier to exercise. We may start off diligent, and we may even stay dedicated for months or years, but as soon as life stress kicks in, we throw in the towel.

Dedication is an important trait to develop for improved mental health through exercise, and it will benefit the rest of our life as well. Dedication implies stick-to-it-ness, tenacity, and diligence. You can feel completely unmotivated yet be so dedicated to your emotional and physical health that you continue to exercise. The best part is that even if you don't feel like a very dedicated exerciser, you can become one. Dedication is a skill that, if practiced, like any other quality, can be learned and cultivated.

Cultivating Dedication

When it comes to cultivating dedication, the first seven keys in this book are a good place to start. Learning about the physical and mental health benefits of exercise can lead to desiring them for yourself, which can become part of your dedication to exercise, especially as you begin to experience them (Key 1). Feeling your confidence grow as you work on embracing self-worth through exercise can help you stay dedicated (Key 2). Family can keep you dedicated (Key 3). Implementing strategies to increase motivation, set achievable goals, and help you alter unhealthy thoughts and beliefs so you can keep moving forward in the spiral of change are each essential parts of long-term dedication (Keys 4 and 5). Learning ways to prevent and overcome roadblocks, and utilizing the FITT principle to create an exercise plan that is relevant and effective for you, are all part of cultivating exercise for mental health dedication.

If you've worked through these first seven keys and have implemented your exercise for mental health plan, but are finding your-self stuck again in some way, then it's time to go back to the drawing board. A core element of dedication is working through the problems that arise and learning to see them as just another part of the process of making change. Remember, as long as you are in the spiral of change, you're making progress. Whether you're moving up or down the spiral doesn't matter as much as staying in the spiral and working towards your goals (Key 5). The only "failure" lies in giving up. You may need to go back to contemplation—re-examine your motivations, core beliefs, or the strategies you thought would work for you. You may need to re-prepare by creating all new goals or by really working on that Pyramid of Self-Worth to build your confidence. You may need to take action again with a fresh exercise for mental health plan. Use the keys in this book like a spiral, and go back or forth according to what you need. There is no one right way to become dedicated to your mental and physical health through exercise. Never be afraid to do it your way, and never be afraid to start over. It's the starting over that forms the foundation of lifelong dedication.

Beyond these seven keys lie a few other tools that can help. Three tools, in particular, I find helpful in cultivating dedication are: 1) creating your exercise for mental health vision; 2) making exercise a habit; and 3) learning and practicing the skills of flour-ishing. Together, these tools can inspire you to live the life you desire—to become confident and diligent in exercise so your mind, body, and spirit can not only be well, but truly and endlessly flourish.

Create Your Exercise for Mental Health Vision

It's one thing to think, "I will stay dedicated to exercise, long-term," or, "I can do anything; my future has great potential." It's another to actually see, strive for, and eventually realize that potential. Cre-ating your exercise for mental health vision is the place to start.

Ponder This . . . Your Vision

When you envision your future, what do you see? In the short-term, can you see yourself acting on your exercise for mental health plan? Can you see yourself growing in confidence, health, and wellness?

Longer-term, can you see yourself remaining active and healthy as you grow older? Can you see yourself raising a healthy, active family, becoming a strength to others after overcoming your own mental health struggles, flourishing in mental and emotional health, or all of these?

Can you see yourself becoming the person you've always desired to be?

Do you know who that person is?

Creating a vision of health and wellness is the first step in realizing your goals. It's the first step in knowing what you're aiming for and recognizing your exercise and mental health potential. Here's how:

1. *Daydream, and dream yourself to sleep.* Dream about all you desire for your emotional, mental, physical, social, and spiritual health. Dream about what your body might feel like, look like, or become. Dream of how your mind will feel—your moods, energy, self-worth, and mental health. Dream of the best possible vision of your family, work, home, and future, and see it clearly in your mind, like a movie.

   At night, as you drift off, instead of thinking of all you have to do the next day, dream yourself to sleep. Envision your best-case exercise and mental health scenario. See how this will positively impact your work, home, and family. See how it will impact and help you realize your future goals, desires, and dreams. Keep that vision clearly in your mind as you fall asleep, again as you wake, and often throughout the day.

2. *Write down what you see.* This is your exercise for mental health vision. It is your motivation and your guide. The more detailed

you can be as you envision your possibilities and write them down, the better. Continue to add to this vision as you work on your exercise for mental health plan and goals. Feel free to alter the vision, or add elements you feel are missing, as you go. And don't be afraid to really go for it. It's your vision, so make it a good one.

3. *Ask yourself, "What will I need to do to achieve this vision?"* Once you have a clear picture of what you hope your future will entail, it's time to back up to the present and ask what it will take to get you there. Be honest as you answer this question. You may find that you need to change your lifestyle if you want to fulfill the vision in your mind. You may find you need to work on your family values, or dig deep and change some underlying beliefs that are preventing you from reaching your vision. Whatever you need to do, write it down. Take as long as you need to create this list of what it will take to get you where you want to be.

4. *Commit to doing the things on your list.* As you see for yourself what your future potential could be, you will likely feel more inspired and motivated to one day see that potential realized. Do you want to achieve that potential you see in your vision? Do you want to live life believing you can do whatever you set your mind to? If so, commit today to doing what it takes.

    Give yourself time on this one. You can't fully commit until you're ready, as the spiral of change reminds us. Be gentle and loving with yourself, and take small steps. You might first commit to *eventually* committing to do the things on your list. Then, when you're ready, you might select one small item and commit to doing that by using Key 4 to set specific, achievable goals. Also, commit to seeking and receiving the help and support you need, so you don't have to do it alone.

5. *Set realistic goals to get you to your desired outcome.* Write down your commitment using the goal-setting strategies and worksheet from Key 4. Set one or two small goals today that will help you get where you want to be tomorrow. They may be the same ones you've already set, or they may be brand new. Either way, remember to break your goals down into small, doable steps. Instead of

setting a goal to "be healthier," set a specific goal, like, "I will improve my nutrition by adding more vegetables, and I will increase my exercise by adding one more 30-minute cardio session each week." Make the goals positive; instead of saying what you will not do, state what you will do. Give yourself a realistic timeline for the goal, and make yourself accountable to someone else.

6. *Get to work.* Take one action today to lead you toward your future exercise for mental health vision. Once you've got that action down, choose another, and so on, until you're living the vision of which you once only dreamed.

Do This . . . Create Your Exercise for Mental Health Vision

Using the steps above, create your vision of exercise and lifelong physical and mental health. Write it down in your journal, notebook, or on your electronic device.

Reflection Questions: Living with Vision

1. What was it like to dream of your future life? Was it easy to see what you desire, or did it take some work to see your vision? Why or why not?

_____

_____

_____

_____

_____

_____

2. How can you remain focused on your vision, to help you stay dedicated to exercise for mental health?

_____

_____

_____

_____

_____

_____

3. What might stand in your way of achieving this vision? How can you prepare now to meet and overcome any challenges that may arise?

_____

_____

_____

_____

_____

Make Exercise a Habit

It's easy to say, "Make exercise a habit," but trust me, I know it's not so easy to do. It's worth the effort, however, because turning a behavior into a habit holds some pretty magical powers. Creating a new habit actually changes our brain in helpful and positive ways. It makes doing that behavior, long-term, much more likely. Exercise is a perfect example. Research shows that those who are able to make a habit of exercise are far more likely to continue exercising for life, and reap far more mental health benefits as a consequence.

In a very real way, exercise habits become automatic, giving us greater mental energy and clarity. Neuroscientists have discovered that the habit-making part of the brain resides in the basal ganglia, which is the area of that brain that's also involved in the creation of emotions, memories, and pattern recognition. On the other hand, decisions, like the decision to exercise or not, are made in the prefrontal cortex—the thinking part of the brain that's also responsible for planning, insight, judgment, and executive functioning. When a decision becomes a habit, that prefrontal cortex is able to essentially go to sleep, meaning that the brain has to work less and less as we develop habits. This is a huge benefit, because it means we save mental energy when we act out of habit, allowing our brain to be fresh for other, more important things.

Charles Duhigg, author of *The Power of Habit*, calls this a "habit loop," which, he says, is a three-part process. Understanding this process can help us create healthy habits—like exercise for mental health. As Duhigg says, "The key to exercising regularly, losing weight, raising exceptional children, becoming more productive, building revolutionary companies and social movements, and achieving success is understanding how habits work" (2012).

Three Components to Creating a Habit

So, how do habits work? According to Duhigg, there are three main components to creating a habit loop: 1) the cue or trigger, 2) the routine, and 3) the reward.

The cue or trigger is what tells your brain to switch into the "automatic mode" of habit when you're doing a behavior. The routine is the behavior itself, which can be physical, mental, or emotional. Our routines can create healthy or unhealthy habits, like exercising or not. The reward is what reinforces the habit loop. When we have an established reward that our brain likes, we are more likely to remember it in the future, and consequently, engage in that behavior. Your reward may be extrinsic, like praise from your trainer or getting to eat a favorite meal or snack after you workout, or may be something that's intrinsic, like noticing how energized, relaxed, or happy you feel when you're done. Either way, rewards are powerful in helping us create a habit.

Chances are, when it comes to exercise, you already have some established habits. You may have some positive habits, like waking up, putting on your jogging clothes and shoes, and heading out the door. The cue in this case is waking up, and the routine is getting dressed and going jogging. The underlying reward may be intrinsic, like remembering, "Even though I'm tired, I'm going jogging, because it will wake me up, get my brain charged, and keep me energized all day long." Or, you may have some not-so-positive habits, like waking up (cue) and thinking, "I really should get up and exercise," and then, laying in bed, stressing over it, until you decide, "I really don't have time, plus I'm way too tired" (routine). This habit loop then involves going to the coffee shop for a double espresso and a chocolate muffin, instead (reward).

Reflection Questions: Your Exercise Habit Loops

1. When it comes to exercise, what are your habit loops? One good way to think of this is by breaking it up into different times of day when you might or might not consider exercising. In the morning, do you have any exercise loops? How about at lunchtime or at work? What about after work, or in the evenings? Try to find your cues, routines, and rewards, and then write them down on the lines below or in your journal or electronic device.

_____

_____

_____

_____

_____

_____

_____

Changing and Creating Habits

Do you have some healthy habit loops for exercise? Do you have any unhealthy habit loops? Either way, for most of us the burning question is, "How do we change the not-so-positive habit loops and create healthier ones?"

Duhigg outlines a framework based on the habit loop components we just identified. In order to change a habit, we first have to understand it. For example, let's say our habit loop is the one mentioned above, where we don't exercise in the morning and instead use coffee and sugar to wake us up and get us out of bed. Sound familiar? For most Americans, I'd say this one has a familiar ring.

Step 1:   *Identify the routine.* The routine, in most cases, is easy to find, because it's the behavior that you want to change. In our case, we want to convert not exercising into exercising. What, exactly, are you habitually doing when you're not exercising? This is your routine. In our example above, we are laying in bed thinking about exercising, and eventually, we replace exercise with coffee and a muffin. Now, we need to investigate a little more. What is our cue for this routine? Is it fatigue? Laziness? Hunger? A sugar or caffeine craving? And what is the reward? Is it sleeping in a little later? Not having to exercise? The caffeine and sugar rush from the coffee and muffin? Getting to see people we like at the coffee shop? A combination of these?

Step 2:   *Experiment with the rewards.* To figure out which of our potential rewards is actually driving the behavior, we need to isolate the various rewards. This may take some time, so be patient and give yourself permission during your experimentation phase to not change. You're trying to understand what you're already doing, so keep doing it, but isolate each potential reward. One day, you might let yourself sleep in during the extra time you'd normally spend analyzing exercise and getting the coffee, and instead, grab a coffee at home. On another day, you might get right out of bed when you first wake up and meet some friends at a café for a healthy breakfast with plenty of social interaction but no caffeine or sugar. As you try different scenarios, you will find which reward is really driving your behavior: avoiding exercise, sleeping in, social interaction, hunger, or caffeine.

One helpful suggestion Duhigg offers is to write down the first three things that come to mind after you test each reward hypothesis. These may be thoughts, feelings, or just the first three words that come to mind. Then, set an alarm on your phone, computer, or watch to go off in 15 to 30 minutes. When it goes off, ask yourself if you still feel the same about the rewards as you did before? Sometimes, being reminded to focus on what you're thinking can help you pay greater attention to and better understand the thoughts and feelings that drive your behavior. Writing down your experience right after is the best way to recall exactly what you were feeling, later, and checking in later is a great way to see if those thoughts and feelings last. It's also a great way to see if your reward actually worked or not (Duhigg, 2012). If, 30 minutes after you slept in or had a healthy breakfast, you're still craving caffeine, then that's a big clue as to which reward is really driving your habit loop.

Step 3: *Isolate the cue.* Cues can be difficult to decipher, because there's so much other information usually present. For instance, do you take a snack break at the same time each day because you're hungry? Or because you're tired? Or because you want to move your stiff body? Or all three? There are countless cues that trigger behaviors; the trick is to decipher which is setting off our habit loop. To do this, Duhigg suggests categorizing potential behaviors ahead of time and then using them to find patterns. He states that almost all habitual cues fall into one of five categories: location, time, emotional state, other people, and proceeding action. In our example of ignoring exercise for the coffee shop, you might write down the following questions to answer when you first wake up:

1. Where are you? (Answer: in bed)
2. What time is it? (Answer: 6:30 A.M.)
3. What's your emotional state? (Answer: tired, unmotivated, stressed)
4. Who else is around? (Answer: no one)
5. What action preceded your urge to ignore exercise and

> head to the coffee shop? (Answer: waking up, looking
> at the clock, thinking of my day, and feeling tired)

Do this for a few days in a row—it will become clear which element is driving your habit. If one element remains fairly consistent, then that's your likely culprit. If, for instance, the time is always the same, but on the next two days you wake up feeling happy and excited for the day, then time is the likely cue, and you'd want to look at perhaps trying to exercise at the end of the day instead. If each day your mood and preceding actions always involve stress and fatigue, then it's probably not the time; no wonder you're turning to caffeine as the easy solution instead of seeking the longer-lasting, powerful effects of exercise.

To Change a Habit, We Need a Plan

If you've established your habit loop's reward, cue, and routine, then it's time to start to change. We change habits by planning for the cues that trigger behavior and then choosing behaviors that provide the reward we're ultimately craving. We discussed how habit turns behaviors that our brain once had to think about into automatic responses; in other words, a habit is a formula that our brain automatically follows. "When I see a cue, I will do a routine in order to get a reward" (Duhigg, 2012). If we want to change this formula, then we have to start making healthier choices, and this involves having a plan.

Create your plan to make exercise a habit using the goal-setting strategies and worksheets in Key 4 and the exercise for mental health plan worksheet in Key 7. Again, make it specific. Include all the elements discussed above: location, time, emotional state, other people, and immediately preceding action. For example, if energy were your main problem, then your plan may be, "I will sleep in and eat a healthy breakfast at home to give me lasting energy in the morning. Then, I will go for a 15-minute walk on my lunch break to give myself an energy boost, eat a protein-rich snack in the afternoon, and take another 15-minute walk after I get home." This is a solid plan to increase energy, let you get a little more sleep, kick the caffeine habit, which actually zaps energy, and ultimately provide you with the long-lasting clarity, effectiveness, and energy you truly desire.

When I first started exercising, it was anything but a habit. My habit was to not exercise; it was to try exercising a few times a month, but get too "busy" or "tired" or "bored" to stick with it. Then, I took my first aerobics class—for college credit. I had to be there in order to get a good grade, and that forced me to start exercising three times a week. At first, I felt stressed in class because I could only do one "boy push-up," and I could barely keep up. But, my cue was having that regular class time and knowing I wanted to keep up a solid grade-point average. At first, my reward was my grade, but over time, my plan to get a good grade in that class made me stick with regular exercise, and by the end of the semester, I enjoyed the aerobics routine and could do 11 regular push-ups. More so, I'd developed a true testimony of how mentally and physically strong and well exercise made me feel.

I kept up my newfound habit of exercising by creating a new plan once the class ended—a plan of walking, doing step aerobics at a local community center, and lifting light weights on alternating days, five days a week. My cue was the specified exercise time when I would workout with friends, and my rewards were the stress release, mental clarity, and increased energy I felt after exercising. Though I started in college by exercising in the evenings, because I couldn't get myself up early enough to do it before class, over the years I developed a new plan, and eventually, a new habit of waking up and exercising first thing in the morning. This has been my habit now for the better part of 20 years.

If you can make a habit of exercise for mental health, you will stay dedicated to exercise, potentially for your entire life. Use the steps above to create a habit of exercise. And as life changes, create new habits. Once again, remind yourself that this may take time. Stay in that spiral of change as you work on your exercise habit plan, going back to the drawing board as often as you need until you're able to turn that daily question, "Do I exercise today? Or not?" into a daily exercise habit.

Learn and Practice the Skills of Flourishing

Flourishing means living to our fullest potential. It is living with meaning, purpose, and joy, contributing, serving, and basking in love. There's so much more out there than just "feeling better," "getting off medication," "looking good," or "losing weight" through exercise. Though these are all valid reasons to exercise, they don't give us the full picture: beyond mental illness lies mental health, and beyond mental health, with the help of exercise, lies flourishing.

We can flourish. We can seek to put the good stuff—joy, love, health—into our lives instead of waiting around for it to just happen. Exercise is one of the best ways to do so.

The Components of Flourishing

To live a flourishing life, we first have to understand flourishing. Dr. Martin Seligman, founder of the positive psychology school of thought, has identified five components of flourishing, which he calls PERMA. PERMA refers to: 1) **P**ositive emotions, 2) **E**ngagement, 3) positive **R**elationships, 4) **M**eaning, and 5) **A**ccomplishment (Seligman, 2012). Together, these five qualities make up a life that is, as I like to say, "better than better" (Hibbert, 2013)—they combine to create a life that flourishes.

Positive Emotions
Considering the impact that exercise has on mood, mental illness, and overall mental wellness, this one is a no-brainer. Exercise is a definite key in creating and maintaining more positive emotions, and conversely, positive emotions make us more likely to exercise. If we want to feel more happiness, joy, love, peace, satisfaction, and yes, even bliss, then we must actively seek these things.

Here are some tips for doing so:

1. *Focus on the positive emotions associated with exercise.* Look for the good in how you feel, and relish it. Remember those truthful affirmations? Remind yourself of the positive experiences and benefits you gain from exercise, and do so often.
2. *Practice gratitude while exercising.* List all your blessings, talents and gifts as you workout. Say a prayer of gratitude as you notice the beauty of nature on a hike, or focus on one thing for which you'll be grateful this day as you finish your stretching. It will bring a deeper sense of appreciation, wonder, and joy, not only to your exercise routine, but to your days, months, and years.

Do This . . . Positive Emotions

1. Before exercising, take a moment to focus on your emotional state. What positive emotions are in you before you exercise? (Even if you feel negative emotions, you can almost always also find at least one positive emotion if you look, such as "excited" to see friends at the gym or "hopeful" that if you take this walk, you'll feel less depressed). Write them down in your journal or notebook.
2. After exercising, take a moment to focus on your emotional state. What positive emotions are in you after you exercise? Write these down, identifying as many as you can (i.e. satisfied, energized, better mood, clearer mind, and so on). Even if it's only one positive emotion, take note. As you exercise more, you will likely feel and identify more positive emotions.

Engagement

Engaging with life in ways that feel useful and helpful, like doing service, sharing talents, and living life with passion, is also linked with exercise for mental health. Simply put, when we exercise, we are engaging more fully in life. We take charge of our physical and mental health, and we witness our body becoming stronger and our mind becoming more relaxed, aware, open, and vibrant. We feel a greater sense of self-confidence when we exercise, and, as we discussed in Key 2, have the potential to feel greater self-worth. All of these help us engage in life with courage, confidence, and love, seek and live out our dreams and passions, and contribute to the greater good.

Here are some tips on ways to engage:

1. *Let exercise make you even better at the things you love to do.* Use exercise to clear your mind, strengthen your energy, and inspire your creativity—this will make you more engaged in life and your specific life pursuits. When working on an important project or creative activity, take exercise breaks. This will clear your mind, give you new ideas, and replenish your body. Remember that study from Key 1? Brainstorming while walking boosts your creativity by 60% over brainstorming while sitting at a desk.

2. *As you exercise, focus on being present and "living in the now."* A big part of engaging fully with life is paying attention to what's right in front of you. Incorporate mindfulness into exercise by using all your senses to take in the world around you. Or, practice mindful relaxation during yoga by getting still and slowing your brain. Focus on breathing, stretching, and doing one rep at a time when you exercise. This will, in turn, help you be more aware in your daily activities, increasing your ability to engage in and experience all that life has to offer.

Reflection Questions: Engagement

1. Do you feel actively engaged with your life? Do you actively seek the good and work hard toward worthy goals? Do you notice the moments that make life great?

Do you try to "live in the now," or is this a struggle for you? Why or why not?

_____

_____

_____

_____

_____

_____

2. How can you use exercise to increase your engagement with the positive things of life? Can you exercise to clear your mind so you're more able to pay attention? Can you practice mindfulness while you exercise? Can you use the mental health benefits of exercise to focus more fully on the good things of life, like family, faith, and friends? Will you? Why or why not?

_____

_____

_____

_____

_____

_____

Positive Relationships

We need positive relationships in order to flourish. This includes relationships with our partner/spouse, children, parents, siblings, grandparents, aunts/uncles, friends, co-workers, acquaintances, and so on. We need to love and to be loved—not only to flourish, but to feel mentally and physically healthy.

When we exercise, we feel better about ourselves and happier. This then helps us interact in more positive, loving ways with family and friends, creating stronger relationships. Additionally, by working out in groups, with a friend, spouse/partner, or child, we can build positive relationships by sharing quality time, a common interest, and encouraging and supporting one another.

Other ways to increase positive relationships through exercise include the following.

1. *Use exercise to increase your social connections and interactions.* Whether you invite friends to workout with you, take an exercise class, or simply talk about your exercise plan with an accountability partner, exercise and social connection go hand in hand. The more you exercise with others, the more connected you become, and the more connected you become, the better your positive relationships, which also leads to better exercise dedication.

2. *Use the self-worth and confidence you receive from exercise to improve relationships.* As you grow in self-worth—through applying The Pyramid of Self-Worth and following through on your exercise goals and plan—you will approach your intimate relationships more confidently and with greater love. Remember two of the components of self-love—letting love in and loving others (Key 2)? Do those. Look for the love in your life and relationships. Then, let it in. Accept the compliment. Say, "thank you," after the kind gesture. Take the hug, and then, return the favor. Focus on receiving love as you also seek to love others more fully, and your relationships will flourish.

Reflection Questions: Positive Relationships

1. How positive are your current relationships? List each important relationship, and then rate how positive it is, from one to five (one being negative, and five being highly positive).

_____

_____

_____

_____

_____

_____

2. Which relationships could use some work right now? Select one or two that you hope to work on, and list below.

_____

_____

_____

3. What can you do to improve this relationship? How can you love more fully, let love in, and use exercise, greater mental health, and self-worth to create more positive relationships in your life?

_____

_____

_____

_____

_____

_____

4. Select one idea, and create a "positive relationships" goal. Use the goal-setting tools/worksheet in Key 4, or write it below. Then, get to work.

_____

_____

_____

Meaning

A life of meaning and purpose is a life that flourishes. Exercise can help us find meaning; and discovering more meaning and purpose in our life can help us stay dedicated to exercise. Exercise helps us feel more meaning in life by strengthening our spiritual connection, sense of self-worth, and mind. In fact, regular exercise can act as a time of reflection on the meaning of life, or it can prepare us to get still and ponder our purpose after we exercise. Exercise can boost our energy, resulting in a greater desire to seek more meaning from life. It can shape a new body and mind so we feel more meaning from the life we're already living.

Conversely, what matters most to us can, and will, shape our exercise and mental health. If, for instance, contribution and service give our life great meaning, then we may look for ways to serve others by involving them in our exercise plan or serving them in more active ways (like doing yard work for an elderly neighbor). True meaning and purpose almost always involve some sense of serving and loving others.

You can increase your sense of meaning and purpose by trying the following.

1. *When exercising, still your thoughts and experience the beauty of the world around you.* Take in all the sights, smells, sounds, and the feel of things as you exercise, especially outdoors. Let it calm your mind, and then let this beauty remind you of the greater meaning and purpose your life holds. Commit to discovering that purpose and fulfilling it.

2. *Ponder what "meaning and purpose" mean to you, and then add more of this to your life.* If family matters most, then create more opportunities to exercise together and spend time as a family. If faith is most important, incorporate your faith and spirituality into your daily exercise routine through prayer, meditation, relaxation, or music.

Ponder This . . . Meaning

What is most meaningful to you? What is your life's purpose? What helps you feel greater meaning and purpose in your life? How can you put more meaning and purpose into your life? Ponder, pray about, or meditate on these things for a time. See what unfolds. When you're ready, write about what you discover in your journal or on your electronic device.

Accomplishment

Above all, regular exercise leads to a sense of accomplishment, and accomplishment is the final element we need in order to flourish.

Accomplishment comes as we commit to exercise, develop goals, and do what we've set out to do. Accomplishment can come as a result of seeing that your body is stronger and healthier as a result of exercise, and that, yes, your mind is, too.

You can increase your sense of accomplishment by considering the following:

1. *Accept, embrace, and celebrate each accomplishment.* When you set a goal, see it as an accomplishment; when you work on building self-worth, see it as an accomplishment; when you reach a goal, feel accomplished, and then celebrate. Reward yourself, reinforcing that goal into a habit. Then, set new goals and accomplishments to achieve.

2. *Never stop seeking growth.* Keep exercise a part of your life. Exercise to enjoy life. Exercise to live a longer life. Exercise to live a happier life. Exercise your whole life long. If you seek growth, then you need to exercise. Exercise is the pathway to true, flourishing growth and accomplishment, in body, mind, spirit, and soul.

Reflection Questions: Accomplishment

1. Do you feel a sense of accomplishment about your exercise, goals, plan, habits, or intentions? Even the smallest bit? If not, why not? What stands in your way of feeling accomplished? If so, what are your accomplishments? Write them below, and be sure to list even the smallest accomplishments.

_____

_____

_____

_____

_____

_____

_____

_____

_____

_____

_____

2. How can you incorporate more exercise for mental health accomplishment into your life? Can you strive to recognize the little steps you take and celebrate them more? Can you pay greater attention to the sense of accomplishment you feel when you suit up, head out the door, and do what you've set out to do? Brainstorm your ideas below, then select one idea and write it into part of your exercise for mental health plan.

_____

_____

_____

_____

_____

_____

3. Revisit all the elements of PERMA, above, and using the activities below each, write down your plan for flourishing. What can you do to increase positive emotion, engagement, relationships, meaning, and achievement in your life?

_____

_____

_____

_____

_____

_____

_____

_____

_____

Flourish in Mental and Physical Health

Dedication is something we can all cultivate, and so is flourishing. We can create and realize our vision for exercise and mental health. We can use that vision to motivate us as we change unhealthy habits and create new, healthy ones. We can then use the exercise habits we create to increase positive emotion, engagement, positive relationships, meaning, and accomplishment in our every day lives. We can use exercise to create a life that flourishes.

Hopefully, reading 8 *Keys to Mental Health Through Exercise* has expanded your view of exercise and mental health. Hopefully, it's helped you see exercise as much more than working out, getting in shape, or even feeling good. Hopefully, these eight keys have helped you reframe exercise as doable—as moving, being active, increasing mental health and wellness, improving family relationships, growing in confidence and self-worth, and having fun while you do so. Hopefully, you now feel the incredible power that exercise can hold in your life—power to *em*power your physical, social, spiritual, emotional, and mental health, and power to take you even beyond health, to flourishing.

Exercise for Mental Health = Exercise for Life

Hopefully, the 8 *Keys to Mental Health Through Exercise* have given you hope—hope that you can create greater mental health through exercise, know the skills and have what it takes, and, should you ever doubt again, know where to turn. You're not alone in this journey. You're part of the exercise for mental health family; and this book, and all of us reading along with you, are right here should you ever need it again.

Choose to exercise. Exercise for mental health. It's not just about exercising to feel better, or look better, or be better. It's about exercising for life—for a longer, happier, and flourishing life.

Reflection Questions: Exercise for Life

1. Now that you've completed this book, which key(s) feel most helpful to you? Why? Which tools, strategies, or skills did you find most helpful or have you utilized most? Why?

_____

_____

_____

_____

_____

_____

2. What areas of exercise and mental health are showing the greatest improvement for you? Why? Which areas still need more work? Why, and what do you intend to do about it?

_____

_____

_____

_____

_____

_____

Visit me at http://www.exercise4mentalhealth.com and join the "Exercise 4 Mental Health Movement!" Register to receive videos, tips, and strategies to keep you exercising all your days. With exercise for mental health, it should be a long, healthy, and happy life.

Center for Disease Control (CDC) Exercise Recommendations, 2011

Generally, for adults, exercise should consist of:

- *Moderate-intensity aerobic exercise*, such as fast walking or cycling: two hours and 30 minutes (or 150 minutes) every week.
- *Strength-training exercises*, such as lifting weights, doing push-ups, or using resistance bands: two or more days each week, working all the major muscle groups.

OR you may choose to do:

- *High-intensity aerobic exercise*, such running, jogging, or swimming laps: one hour and 15 minutes (75 minutes) a week, along with the recommended two or more days of strength-training exercises.

OR you may choose to do:

- A mix of the two options above.

For even greater physical and mental health benefits, and if cleared by your doctor, you may opt to:

- *Increase your cardiovascular activity*, per week, to either: 300

minutes of moderate-intensity activity plus two or more days of strength training, or 150 minutes of high-intensity cardio plus strength training, or a mix of these two options.

These recommendations focus on making exercise part of a weekly routine, not just a daily one, which implies that if you skip a day (or two, or three), it doesn't mean you've failed. You still have several other days to meet your weekly exercise goals.

The Office of Disease Prevention and Health Promotion (ODPHP, 2008) offers further exercise recommendations, for each life phase:

- *Children and adolescents:* Up to one hour, or even more, of physical activity per day, including aerobic activities (i.e. playing tag, sports, and so on) and muscle- and bone-strengthening activities that are age appropriate. Bone-strengthening activities refer to anything that produces a force on the bones. This force strengthens and creates bone growth. Sports like basketball or tennis, running and jumping rope, and even playing hopscotch can all strengthen bones. Remember that activity choices will vary among children, and they should be age appropriate. What looks like "play" or "goofing around" to adults is actually exercise for kids. Encourage them to get up, get out, and get moving—in whatever ways they enjoy.
- *Adults:* The biggest key for adults is to avoid inactivity. As we've discussed in previous chapters, too many of us give up physical activity when we reach adulthood. Remember that exercise consists of anything that gets you up and moving. Total exercise time includes: work-related movement—taking the stairs three times a day or doing a walking meeting; family-related movement—playing tag or soccer with your kids or going for a family bike ride; home-related movement—vigorous house-cleaning or gardening; and social movement—going for a hike with friends.
- *Older Adults:* Since there tends to be greater diversity in exercise ability as we get older—with some in peak condition and others

struggling with chronic health problems and loss of physical fitness—the most important thing is to stay active, to exercise for life your whole life long. First, keep in touch with your doctor to obtain fitness recommendations and clearance for exercise. Then, focus on staying as physically active as possible for your situation. If you're unable to do the recommended 150 minutes of moderate-intensity or 75 minutes of high-intensity exercise per week, that's okay. Just do what you can. Strength-training activities (i.e. lifting weights, using resistance bands) are important when we're older, to keep muscle mass and increase bone density, but we need to be cautious to prevent injury. Use lighter weights with more repetitions to start. You can even do upper body exercises with light weights while sitting in a chair. Make sure to also incorporate balance (i.e. backwards walking, standing from a sitting position) and flexibility (i.e. yoga, stretching) exercises, which are especially helpful as we grow older.

Mental Health Across the Lifespan: The Facts

Childhood Mental Health

Mental health issues and disorders are more common in children than most people think:

- Fifteen million children may currently be diagnosed with a mental health disorder.
- Even more children are at high risk of developing a mental illness in the future, thanks to genetic, family, school, friends, and community factors (APA, 2015).
- Childhood mental disorders appear to be on the rise. One study revealed that pediatric visits resulting in a mental health diagnosis rose from 8.1% in 2010 to 10.5% in 2013, a rise of 29% (Sung, 2013).
- The most common childhood mental health diagnoses include: Attention-Deficit/Hyperactivity Disorder (ADHD), 6.8% of kids age 3 to 17; behavioral or conduct problems, 3.5%; anxiety disorders, 3%; Depression, 2.1%, and autism-spectrum disorders, 1.1% (Perou et al., 2013).
- While childhood rates for ADHD and autism are higher for boys, girls have higher rates of anxiety, depression, and eating disorders (Sung, 2013).
- Depression and anxiety often occur together in children, and those affected tend to have recurring episodes as they grow older.

- As children age, depression becomes more prevalent, and it's not always easy for parents and caregivers to identify. In grade school, symptoms of depression may appear more physical, with complaints of aches and pains. Rather than saying, "I'm depressed," children may struggle at school, have difficulty with friends or family, and not know how to talk about what they're feeling (NAMI, 2014). Episodes of childhood depression tend to last around six to nine months, but can become chronic without treatment.
- Childhood mental health disorders also tend to co-occur with health and medical conditions that can affect treatment methods and adherence, and are associated with later substance abuse, risky sexual behaviors, criminal acts, lower educational achievement, and less successful functioning in work, family, and parenting (Perou, 2013).

Teen Mental Health and Exercise

Research on teen mental health shows that:

- depression risk increases as children move into adolescence and grow older; in fact, it's estimated that 11% of teens have a depressive disorder by age 18 (NIMH, 2015a). Over half of those with depression in adolescence will experience a recurring depressive episode within the next seven years (NIMH 2015-1). Untreated mental illness in teens can often develop into long-term mental illness.
- though depression rates for boys and girls are equal in younger childhood, by adolescence, girls are depressed almost twice as much as boys, and it stays that way throughout the lifespan (Sung, 2013). This points to several factors, including the biological influence of changing hormone levels in teenage girls, and the differences between how girls and boys process emotional stress.
- depression symptoms in teens may include anger, irritability, or hostility, low self-esteem, extreme sensitivity to failure or rejection, and relationship issues, isolation, low energy, hopelessness,

crying, complaints of physical illness (like stomach or head-aches), major changes in sleep or appetite, lack of interest in activities once enjoyed, hopelessness, and even thoughts of sui-cide (NAMI, 2014). It's important for caregivers to understand and help identify these symptoms to get teens the support and treatment they need.

- Depressed teens tend to cope through drugs or alcohol, aggres-sion, slacking off in school, or sometimes, running away (NAMI, 2014). They may seem fine on the outside, but inside, they're feeling empty, isolated, and hopeless.

- It's estimated that 4.7% of youth ages 12 to17 reported an illicit drug use and 4.2% were diagnosed with an alcohol abuse disor-der in the past year, while 2.8% were dependent on cigarettes in the past month (Perou et al., 2013).

- According to one study, 8% of teens reported greater than or equal to 14 "mentally unhealthy days" in the past month (Perou et al., 2013), and in 2010, the adolescent suicide rate was 4.5 suicides per 100,000 people (Perou et al., 2013).

- Lack of exercise, lack of sleep, and too much media also affect mental health. Social media can have a particularly powerful effect on self-worth and body image, with bullying and popular-ity contests giving teens unrealistic ideas about how to be accepted and liked online.

- Many at-risk teens fall under the radar. One European study of 12,395 adolescents from 11 countries found that 13% of teens were considered "high risk" for anxiety, depression, and suicidal-ity, since these teens engaged in high levels of risky behaviors, like drugs and alcohol; 58% were considered "low risk;" and the researchers were surprised to find that 29% of teens made up a new category they called "invisible risk." The teens in the invisi-ble risk group had high media use, low sleep, and were seden-tary, yet they showed similar levels of anxiety, depression, and suicidal ideation to the high-risk group (Carli et al., 2014).

- Risk behaviors and mental illness are relatively common among teens, and these risk behaviors and symptoms increase with age (Carli et al., 2014). The most common risk factors for boys are drug and alcohol use, while lack of activity and reduced sleep are more common among girls.

Young Adult Mental Health and Exercise

As we move into our early- to mid-twenties, we get to see what our adult body and mind are all about. The brain is now fully formed, and we are immersed in discovering our path in life, understanding our identity as an adult, and working on who we want to be. Young adult life is dynamic and varied, as we navigate schooling, career choices, self-responsibility and finances, developing family relationships, dating, and maybe even getting married. Yet, it's also a critical time for mental health, a time when we are most vulnerable to the onset of mental illness.

- Three of four people diagnosed with mental illness showed signs before the age of 24 (USDHHS, 2015). In fact, schizophrenia, bipolar disorder, and major depressive disorder most commonly appear in the late teens or early twenties. It's believed the stress of young adult life may trigger the onset of these and other disorders that may have been laying dormant. Stressors such as going to college, caring for oneself, and living away from family can contribute to the onset of mental illness (SAMHSA, 2014).

- Drug and alcohol use can also trigger the onset of mental illness, especially with hallucinogens like marijuana or cocaine. Young adults may turn to alcohol or drug use to cope with mental stress or illness, but these substances typically lead to far more problems, including a substance abuse or dependence disorder.

- One in five young adults (18 to 25 years old) had a mental illness in the past year, based on combined data from 2010 to 2012; 3.9% suffered from a serious mental illness, and 6.4% of young adults had co-occurring mental illness and substance use disorder. Young adults suffering from mental illness report poorer quality of life (SAMHSA, 2014).

- It's estimated that 66.6% of young adults with mental illness do

not receive treatment or help, and 47% of those with serious
mental illness go untreated.

- Early intervention is crucial to help young adults adjust to their
new life roles and set them up with the skills and outlook they
need for a life of success and happiness.

Childbearing Years Mental Health and Exercise

The years of childbearing and parenting young children can be
some of the most challenging. For one, the hormonal shifts that
accompany pregnancy and childbirth can throw many women
into a struggle with a perinatal mood or anxiety disorder, like postpartum depression, and this can significantly impact her partner/
spouse, children, and entire family. Men also experience shifts in
emotional functioning after a baby is born and can develop paternal postnatal depression (PPND).

Lack of sleep is another issue that's common in the childbearing years, with most parents fighting off fatigue and exhaustion on
a daily basis. Time is suddenly consumed with caregiving, providing for, and spending time with children and family, in addition to
previous work and personal responsibilities. It's a season of high
stress and no sleep that can take its toll on a mother or father's
mental health.

To better understand the unique mental health needs of the
childbearing years, let's look at the facts:

- Pregnancy and the first year postpartum are a particularly vulnerable time in a woman's life. A woman is 30 times more likely to
experience a psychotic episode in the days immediately following childbirth than any other time in her life. This shows just
how stressful and challenging the childbearing years can be.
- Postpartum mental health falls on a spectrum, with disorders
ranging from mild to severe. On the mild end, up to 80% of
women will experience some change in their emotional health
during or after childbirth. This is most commonly referred to as

"The Baby Blues," and typically goes away without treatment. In the middle of the spectrum, we see depression and anxiety disorders. Up to 15% of women will have depression in pregnancy, and as many as one in five will experience postpartum depression. Approximately 6% of pregnant and 10% of postpartum women suffer from an anxiety disorder, while 3-5% experience pregnancy/postpartum OCD, and 1-6% experience postpartum posttraumatic PTSD (PSI, 2014). On the severe end of the spectrum, 1 in 1000 women will experience postpartum psychosis, a serious and potentially life-threatening mental illness that requires immediate treatment to protect both mother and baby.

- Together, these perinatal mood/anxiety disorders have been called the most common complication associated with childbirth.
- If untreated, pregnancy/postpartum mental illness can become chronic. Maternal depression affects approximately 10% of mothers, after the postpartum period, each year. Only about half seek and receive treatment, and it is estimated that at least 1 in 10 American children has a depressed mother in any given year (Ertel at al., 2011). Maternal depression is one of the strongest predictors of future behavioral and cognitive problems in the developing child (Canadian Pediatric Society, 2004).
- It's estimated as many as 10% of fathers worldwide, and 14% in the United States, experience PPND (Paulson & Bazemore, 2010), which can also become chronic if untreated. Some estimate these numbers to be even higher, considering many do not discuss their symptoms nor reach out for help.
- About half of men who have depressed partners are also depressed. When both parents are depressed, it can have a significant impact on parenting, bonding, and the overall development and well-being of the baby and other children.

Middle Age Mental Health and Exercise

Middle age can be a time of great physical and emotional change. Sending kids off to college, "empty nest" syndrome, the end or beginning of careers, and relationship changes can all add to the exhilaration, and stress, of this season of life. For many, middle age is a time of financial security and a sense of mastery and competence, while for others, these years can be a time of financial stress, facing debt while also supporting college-aged children or aging parents. Some experience the middle years as a time of freedom that boosts career options and relationships, while other face regret and sorrow over stale marriages and stalled careers. Add to this caring for aging parents or dealing with your own changing body or declining health, and it can be a stressful and vulnerable time for mental health.

Women face an especially unique set of circumstances in middle age, as their menstrual cycle begins to come to a halt. *Perimenopause* refers to the months, or years, leading up to menopause, or the cessation of one's menstrual cycle. This phase of life often brings physical and emotional symptoms that can severely disturb a woman's mental health. Relationships may also change through menopause, and it can be one of the toughest times in a couple's relationship.

For men, "mid-life crisis" is common, though most experts agree it's not so much a crisis as a time of major life transition. While a "mid-life crisis" can occur in women, especially as their hormones shift and alter, men are more likely to experience mental health symptoms related to their changing careers and bodies. Many men have a hard time with the physical changes of middle age and wonder, "Whose body is this, anyway?" Others may feel their career path didn't pan out as they'd hoped. Men are less likely to build supportive social networks and share their troubles, and more likely to indulge in heavy drinking to cope. Suicide is thus another common issue in middle-aged men (Doheny, 2008).

Knowing the facts about middle life mental health can help everyone prepare:

- The average age for menopause in the United States is 45 to 55, and perimenopause can last for months or as many as 10 years. Each year, 1.3 million women reach menopause in the United

States, and it's estimated 20% of these have depression at some point during the process (Gramann, 2012).

- While many navigate perimenopause with no mood symptoms, studies show an increased risk of depression in perimenopausal women that decreases after menopause (NIMH, 2015c). This risk is the same even for women with no previous mental illness history (Freeman et al., 2006; Cohen et al., 2006). The perimenopausal years also put women at risk for greater anxiety, panic disorder, and OCD, and can exacerbate symptoms of bipolar disorder, especially depressive episodes (Gramann, 2012). This points, once more, to the great part hormones play in women's mental health.

- While schizophrenia typically manifests itself in men and women in young adulthood, middle age presents a second peak in the onset of schizophrenia for women aged 45 to 50, and some women experience a worsening of schizophrenia during perimenopause, again suggesting the role of hormones in mental illness (Gramann, 2012).

- Insomnia is also common during the menopausal transition, with 40-50% of women experiencing sleep disturbances. Women suffering from insomnia are also more likely to report symptoms of anxiety, tension, stress, and depression (Gramann, 2012).

- While women are three times more likely to attempt suicide than men, men are four times more likely to die by suicide than women (NAMI, 2015). Men tend to employ more lethal means, with nearly 60% of male suicides using a firearm, and men are also more likely to drink heavily when distressed. It's estimated that 90% of those who die by suicide have some form of mental illness or substance abuse disorder (Fields, 2010).

- Suicide rates are actually highest among middle-aged men; in fact, middle-aged white men have the highest suicide rates of any group (American Foundation for Suicide Prevention [AFSP], 2015; Bilsker & White, 2011). "Women seek help, men die," one 1990 medical journal stated, and though it's certainly an exaggeration, there is definitely some truth to it (Fields, 2010).

The Golden Years—Exercise for Mental Health

As life winds down, the years of old age carry with them many changes. The death of a spouse, family, and loved ones is common as we grow older, and grief can be a constant companion. Declining health and chronic illness can also have a big impact in later life. However, for many, the years of retirement are considered "the golden years," and certainly, there is much life to be lived as we grow old.

Depression is fairly common in old age, and many believe it to be a "normal" part of aging. It's not. Depression may be overlooked because older adults may not be as willing to discuss or treat symptoms of sadness or grief. Doctors may also be less likely to spot depression, often attributing it to other physical conditions or "normal" aging.

While depression is not a normal part of aging, for many, cognitive decline is, and over time, many may suffer from restricted blood flow to the body, including the brain. This can lead to depression-like symptoms, and may also put people afflicted at greater risk for heart disease or stroke (NIMH, 2015b).

Here are the facts:

- It's estimated that seven million Americans over age 65 suffer from depression (Kerr, 2012). Unfortunately, depression in the elderly often goes unnoticed or is mistaken for some other condition, and therefore, it often goes untreated (Kerr, 2012).
- Older women experience depression more than men, but depression rates significantly decline in women after menopause (NIMH, 2015c). Rates of depression are significantly lower for elderly living on their own (1-5%) versus living in the hospital (14%) or in a nursing home (29-52%) (Kerr, 2012).
- It's estimated as many as 90% of the elderly suffering from depression do not receive adequate care, and 78% receive no treatment at all (Kerr, 2012). Those in this age group are most likely to "handle it themselves," and many do not see depression as a health condition (Mental Health America [MHA], 2015).

- The suicide rate for those 85 years and older is the second highest of any age group, with men at highest risk (AFSP, 2015). This is a terrible tragedy, with so many feeling lost and alone at the end of life.
- It is common in the elderly for depression to be triggered by other illnesses, like Parkinson's, Alzheimer's, heart disease, cancer, and arthritis (MHA, 2015). Physical and mental health are especially intertwined in the golden years.
- Widowhood is another factor that can impact mental health in later years. It's estimated that 15-30% of widows/widowers meet the criteria for clinical depression in the first year (Sasson & Umberson, 2013), and many more exhibit subclinical depression (Carr & Utz, 2001). Half of these remain depressed after one year (van Grootheest et al., 1999). Women are at greater risk of early widowhood, and men tend to remarry more often than women after the death of a spouse. Widowhood earlier in life is associated with higher rates of depression and poorer adjustment than later widowhood (Sasson & Umberson, 2013), though there is some variation in the research. Overall, women seem to adjust to widowhood more readily than men, while older men who remain alone are at a higher risk of depression than widowed women or men who remarry (van Grootheest et al., 1999).
- Cognitive decline is another significant issue in older years. One in three seniors die with Alzheimer's or another form of dementia, and it's estimated that by 2050, the number of those with Alzheimer's may triple, from five million to as many as 16 million (Alzheimer's Association, 2015a).
- For many, however, the years after menopause (for women) and retirement are filled with new learning and experiences, grandchildren and family, and a renewal of life—especially for those who remain physically active.

References

Abrantes, A.M., Strong, D.R., Cohn, A., Cameron, A.Y., Greenberg, B.D., Mancebo, M.C., & Brown, R.A. (2009). Acute changes in obsessions and compulsions following moderate-intensity aerobic exercise among patients with obsessive-compulsive disorder. *Journal of Anxiety Disorders*, 23(7), 923-927.

Alcoholrehab.com. (2015). *Exercise an effective treatment in rehab: physical fitness can help in early recovery.* Accessed April 4, 2015. Retrieved from http://alcoholrehab.com/alcoholism/exercise-for -alcohol-rehab-treatment/

Alzheimer's Association. (2015a). *Alzheimer's facts and figures.* Accessed Feb. 2, 2015. Retrieved from http://www.alz.org/alzheim ers_disease_facts_and_figures.asp

Alzheimer's Association. (2015b). *Stay physically active.* Accessed Feb. 2, 2015. Retrieved from http://www.alz.org/we_can_help_stay_phys- ically_active.asp

American Foundation for Suicide Prevention [AFSP]. (2015). *Facts and figures.* Accessed January 15, 2015. Retrieved from https://www .afsp.org/understanding-suicide/facts-and-figures

American Heart Association. (Nov. 13, 2014). *The AHA's recommenda- tions for physical activity in children.* Accessed Jan. 28, 2015. Retrieved from http://www.heart.org/HEARTORG/GettingHealthy/ HealthierKids/ActivitiesforKids/The-AHAs-Recommendations-for -Physical-Activity-in-Children_UCM_304053_Article.jsp

American Institute of Stress (AIS). (n.d.) *Stress is killing you.* Accessed Jan. 7, 2015. Retrieved from http://www.stress.org/stress-is-killing-you/

American Psychological Association. *Children's mental health.* Accessed Jan. 23, 2015. Retrieved from http://www.apa.org/pi/families/chil dren-mental-health.aspx

American Society of Addiction Medicine. (April 9, 2011). *Definition of addiction: Public policy statement.* Accessed June 2, 2015. Retrieved from http://www.asam.org/for-the-public/definition-of-addiction

Andel, R., Crowe, M., Pederson, N.L., Fratiglioni, L., Johansson, B., &

Gatz, M. (2008). Physical exercise at midlife and risk of dementia three decades later: A population-based study of Swedish twins. *The Journals of Gerontology*, Series A, 63(1), 62-66.

Anxiety and Depression Association of America [ADAA]. (2014). *Facts and Statistics*. Accessed June 8, 2015. Retrieved from http://www.adaa.org/about-adaa/press-room/facts-statistics

Arizona Postpartum Wellness Coalition. (2005). *Perinatal mood and anxiety disorders: assessment & treatment*. (2-day certificate of completion course). AZ.

Aruajo, C.G. & Stein, R. (Aug. 10, 2015). *Leisure time physical activity and mortality: it is time to fill the prescription — more activity for adults*. Accessed September 14, 2015. Retrieved from http://www.acc.org/latest-in-cardiology/articles/2015/08/07/12/01/leisure-time-physical-activity-and-mortality?w_nav=TI

Babyak, M., Blumenthal, J.A., Herman, S., Khatri, P., et al. (2000). Exercise treatment for major depression: maintenance of therapeutic benefit at 10 months. *Psychosomatic Medicine*, 62(5), 633-8.

Baxter, A.J., Scott, K.M., Vos, T., & Whiteford, H.A. (2013). Global prevalence of anxiety disorders: A systematic review and meta-regression. *Psychological Medicine*, 43(5), 897-910.

Belloc, N.B. & Breslow, L. (1972). Relationship of physical health status and health practices. *Preventive Medicine*, 1(3), 409-21.

Beretsky, S. (April 15, 2011). *When Exercise Feels Just Like a Panic Attack*. Accessed June 22, 2015. http://psychcentral.com/blog/archives/2011/04/14/when-physical-exercise-feels-just-like-a-panic-attack/

Bergland, C. (2013). *Cortisol: why "the stress hormone" is public enemy no. 1*. Accessed Setpember 11, 2015. Retrieved from https://www.psychologytoday.com/blog/the-athletes-way/201301/cortisol-why-the-stress-hormone-is-public-enemy-no-1

Bernard, P. & Ninot, G. (2012). Benefits of exercise for people with schizophrenia: A systematic review. *Encephale*, 38(4), 280-7.

Bhargava, H.D. (reviewed by). (2014). *5 simple, fun ideas for family fitness*. Accessed June 4, 2015. Retrieved from http://www.webmd.com/parenting/raising-fit-kids/move/family-fitness-ideas

Biddle, S.J. & Asare, M. (2011). Physical activity and mental health in children and adolescents: A review of reviews. *British Journal of Sports Medicine*, 45, 886-895.

Biddle, S.J. & Fox, K.R. (1989). Exercise and health psychology: Emerging relationships. *British Journal of Medical Psychology*, 62, 205-216.

Blair, S. (1995). Exercise prescription for health. *Quest*, 47, 338-353.

Blisker, D. & White, J. (2011). The silent epidemic of male suicide. *British Columbia Medical Journal*, 52(10), 529-534.

Blumenthal, J.A., Babyak, M.A., Doraiswamay, M., Watkins, L., Hoffman, B.M., Barbour, K.A., et al. (2007). Exercise and pharmacotherapy in the treatment of major depressive disorder. *Psychosomatic Medicine*, 69, 587-596.

Branden, N. (1995). *The six pillars of self-esteem: The definitive work on self-esteem by the leading pioneer in the field.* Bantam Books: New York, NY.

Brooks, A., Bandelow, B., Pekrun, G., Meyer, T., et al. (1998). Comparison of aerobic exercise, clomipramine, and placebo in the treatment of panic disorder. *American Journal of Psychiatry*, 155(5), 603-9.

Brown, S. (2008). *Play is more than just fun.* [video] TedTalks. Accessed Feb. 24, 2015. http://www.ted.com/talks/stuart_brown_says_play_is_more_than_fun_it_s_vital?language=en#t-26377

Brustad, R.J. (1993) Who will go out and play? Parental and psychological influences on children's attraction to physical activity. *Pediatric Exercise Science*, 5(3), 210-223.

Brustad, R.J. (2010). The role of the family in promoting physical activity. *President's Council on Physical Fitness & Sports Research Digest*, 10(3), 1-8.

Canadian Pediatric Society. (2004). Maternal depression and child development. *Pediatric Child Health*, 9(8), 575–583.

Carli, V. et al. (2014). A newly identified group of adolescents at invisible risk for psychopathology and suicidal behavior: Findings from the SEYLE study. *World Psychiatry*, 13(1), 78-86.

Carr, D. & Utz, R. (2001). Late-life widowhood in the United States: New directions in research and theory. *Ageing International*, 27(65).

Cash, H., Rae, C.D., Steel, A.H., & Winklerb, A. (2012). Current psychiatry reviews, 8(4), 292-298.

Centers for Disease Control and Prevention. (2011). *How much physical activity do adults need?* Accessed Dec. 13, 2014. Retrieved from http://www.cdc.gov/physicalactivity/everyone/guidelines/adults.html

Centers for Disease Control and Prevention. (2015). *CDC behavioral risk factor surveillance survey.* Accessed Feb. 7, 2015. Retrieved from http://www.cdc.gov/brfss/

Chouloff, F. (1994). Influence of physical exercise on 5-HT1A receptor and anxiety-related behaviors. *Neuroscience Letters*, 176(2), 226-230.

Chouloff, F. (1997). The serotonin hypothesis. In W.P. Morgan (Ed.), *Physical Activity and Mental Health*. Taylor and Francis: Washington, D.C., 179-98.

Clayton, R. (2014). How regular exercise helps you balance work & family. *Harvard Business Review*. Accessed Feb. 22, 2015. Retrieved from https://hbr.org/2014/01/how-regular-exercise-helps-you-balance-work-and-family

Cohen, G.E. & Shamus, E. (2009). Depressed, low self-esteem? What can exercise do for you? *The Internet Journal of Allied Sciences and Practices*, (7)2, 1-5.

Cohen L., Altshuler L., Harlow B., Nonacs R., Newport DJ, Viguera A., Suri R., Burt V., Hendrick A.M., Loughead A., Vitonis A.F., Stowe Z. (2006). Relapse of major depression during pregnancy in women who maintain or discontinue antidepressant treatment. *Journal of the American Medical Association*, 295(5), 499-507.

Cook, B., Hausenblas, H., Tuccitto, D., Giacobbi, G.R. (2011). Eating disorders and exercise: A structural equation modeling analysis of a conceptual model. *Eur. Eat. Disorders Rev.*, 19, 216–225.

Covey, S. (2013). *The seven habits of highly effective people: Powerful lessons in personal change*. New York: Simon & Schuster.

Craft, L.L. & Perna, F.M. (2004). The benefits of exercise for the clinically depressed. *Primary Care Companion to the Journal of Clinical Psychiatry*, 6(3), 104-111.

Crocker, J. (2002). The costs of seeking self-esteem. *Journal of Social Issues*, 58(3), 597-615.

Daly, A.J., Macarthur, C., & Winter, H. (2007). The role of exercise in treating postpartum depression: A review of the literature. *Journal of Midwifery and Women's Health*, 52(1), 56-62.

Depression and Bipolar Support Alliance. (2015). *Depression statistics*. Accessed Jan. 12, 2015. Retrieved from http://www.dbsalliance.org/site/PageServer?pagename=education_statistics_depression

Diener, E. (1984). Subjective well-being. *Psychological Bulletin*, 95, 542-575.

Doheny, K. (2008). *Midlife crisis: Transition or depression?* Accessed Jan. 31, 2015. Retrieved from http://www.webmd.com/depression/features/midlife-crisis-opportunity

Driver, H.S. and Taylor, S.R. (2000). Exercise and sleep. *Sleep Medicine Reviews*, 4(4), 387–402.

Duhigg, C. (2012). *The power of habit: Why we do what we do in life and business*. New York: Random House.

Duncan, S.C., Duncan, T.E., Strycker, L.A. (2005). Sources and types of social support in youth physical activity. *Health Psychology*, 24(1), 3-10.

Durden-Smith, J. (1978). A chemical cure for madness. *Quest*, 2, 31-36.

Dzewaltowski, D.A., Geller, K.S., Rosenkranz, R.R., Karteroliotis, K. (2010). Children's self-efficacy and proxy efficacy for after-school physical activity. *Psychology of Sports and Exercise*, 11(1), 100-106.

Eaton, W.W., Shao, H., Nestadt, G., Lee, J.B., Bienvenu, O.J., & Zandi, P. (2008). Population-based study of first onset of chronicity in major depressive disorder. *Archives of General Psychiatry*, 65, 513-520.

Ekeland E., Heian F., Hagen, K.B., Abbott, J.M., & Nordheim, L. (2004). Exercise to improve self-esteem in children and young people. *Cochrane Database of Systematic Reviews*, (1): CD003683.

Ertel, K.A., Rich-Edwards, J.W., & Koenen, K.C. (2011). Maternal depression in the United States: Nationally representative rates and risks. *J Women's Health*, 20(11), 1609–1617.

Faulkner, B. & Biddle, S. (1999). Exercise as an adjunct treatment for schizophrenia: A review of the literature. *Journal of Mental Health*, 3(5), 441-457.

Fields, D. (2010). *Middle-age suicide*. Accessed Feb. 4, 2015. Retrieved from http://goodmenproject.com/featured-content/middle-age-sui cide/

Fogarty M, Happell B, & Pinikahana J. (2004). The benefits of an exercise program for people with schizophrenia: A pilot study. *Psychiatric Rehabilitation Journal*, 28, 173–176.

Fox, K. (2000). The effects of exercise on self-esteem & self-perceptions. *Physical Activity & Psychological Well-Being*; Biddle, S., Fox, K., & Boutcher, S. (Eds.). Psychology Press, 88-98.

Freeman E.W., Sammel M.D., Lin H., Nelson D.B. (2006). Associations of hormones and menopausal status with depressed mood in women with no history of depression. *Archives of General Psychiatry*, 63(4), 375-382.

Fritz, R. (1989). *Path of Least Resistance: Learning to become the creative force in your own life*. New York, NY: Ballantine Books.

Fulton, J.D., Shisler, J.L., Yore, M.M., Caspersen, C.J. (2006). Active transportation to school: Findings from a national survey. *Research Quarterly for Exercise and Sport*, 76(3), 352-357.

Galvin, R., Cusack, T., O'Grady, E., Murphy, T.B., & Stokes, E. (2011).

Family-mediated exercise intervention (FAME): Evaluation of a novel form of exercise delivery after stroke. *Stroke*, 42, 681-686.

Garber, C.E., Blissmer, B., Deschenes, M.R., Franklin, B.A., Lamonte, M.J., Lee, I., Nieman, D.C., & Swain, D.P. (2011). Quantity and quality of exercise for developing and maintaining cardiorespiratory, musculoskeletal, and neuromotor fitness in apparently healthy adults: Guidance for prescribing exercise. *Medicine and Science in Sports and Exercise*, 43(7), 1334-1359.

Gerber, M., Brand, S., Elliot, C., Holsboer-Trachsler, E., Puhse, U., & Beck, J. (2013). Aerobic exercise training and burnout: A pilot study with male participants suffering from burnout. *BMC Research Notes*, 2013, 6:78.

Gillen, J.B., Percival, M.E., Skelly, L.E., Martin, B.J., Tan, R.B., et al. (2014). Three minutes of all-out intermittent exercise per week increases skeletal muscle oxidative capacity and improves cardio-metabolic health. *PLoS One*, 9(11): e111489.

Goldberg, J. (reviewed by). (August 21, 2014). *Electroconvulsive therapy and other depression treatments*. Accessed September 12, 2015. Retrieved from http://www.webmd.com/depression/guide/electro convulsive-therapy

Goodreads. (2015). *Benjamin Franklin: Quotable quote*. Accessed September 11, 2015. Retrieved from http://www.goodreads.com/quotes/1220489-energy-and-persistence-conquer-all-things

Goodwin, R.D. (2003). Association between physical activity and mental disorders among adults in the United States. *Preventive Medicine*, 36, 689-703.

Gorczynski, P. & Faulkner, G. (2010). Exercise therapy for schizophrenia. *Cochrane Database Syst Rev*, 12(5).

Gordon, J. (2001). *Comprehensive cancer care: Integrating alternative, complementary, and conventional therapies*. Cambridge, MA: Perseus Publishing

Gramann, S. (April, 2012). *Menopause & mood disorders*. Accessed Feb. 5, 2015. Retrieved from http://emedicine.medscape.com/article/295382-overview.

Griffin, S.J., and Trinder, J. (1978) Physical fitness, exercise, and human sleep. *Psychophysiology*, 15(5), 447-50.

Gutin, B. (1966). Effect of increase in physical fitness on mental ability following physical and mental stress. *Research Quarterly*, 37(2), 211-20.

Hamer, M., Sabia, S., Batty, G.D., Shipley, M.J., Tabak, A.G., Singh-

Manoux, A., et al. (2012). Physical activity and inflammatory markers over 10 years: Follow-up in men and women from the Whitehall II cohort study. *Circulation, 126*(8), 928-33.

Hayden, J.A., van Tulder, M.W., Malmivaara, A., & Koes, B.W. (2005). Exercise therapy for treatment of non-specific low back pain. *Cochrane Database of Systematic Reviews, 20(3),* CD000335.

Harvard Health Publications. (2015). *What's the best exercise plan for me?* Accessed Feb. 15, 2015. Retrieved from http://www.helpguide .org/harvard/whats-the-best-exercise-plan-for-me.htm

Helmrich, S. P., Ragland, D.R., Leung, R.W., & Paffenbarger, R.S. Jr. (1991). Physical activity and reduced occurrence of non-insulin-dependent diabetes mellitus. *New England Journal of Medicine,* 325(3), 147-52.

Herring, M.P., Jacob, M.L., Subeg, C., Dishman, R.K., & O'Connor, P.J. (2012). Feasibility of exercise training for the short-term treatment of generalized anxiety disorder: a randomized controlled trial. *Psychotherapy and Psychosomatics,* 81, 21-28.

Hibbert, C. (2013). *This is how we grow: A psychologist's memoir of loss, motherhood, and discovering self-worth and joy, one season at a time.* Flagstaff, AZ: Oracle Folio.

Hibbert, C. (2015). *Who am I without you? 52 ways to rebuild self-esteem after a breakup.* Ontario, CA: New Harbinger Publications.

Huberty, J.L., Ransdell, L.B., Sidman, C., Flohr, J.A., Shultz, B., Grosshans, O., & Durrant, L. (2008). Explaining long-term exercise adherence in women who complete a structured exercise program. *Research Quarterly for Exercise and Support,* (79)3, 374-384.

Hull, E.E., Rofey, D.L., Robertson, R.J., Nagle, E.F., Otto A.D., & Aaron, D.J. (2010). Influence of marriage and parenthood on physical activity: A 2-year prospective analysis. *J Phys Act Health,* 7(5), 577-583.

Hunter, G.R., McCarthy, J.P., Bamman, M.M. (2004). Effects of resistance training on older adults. *Sports Medicine,* 34, 329-348.

Iannotti, R.J. & Wang, J. (2013). Patterns of physical activity, sedentary behavior, and diet in U.S. adolescents. *Journal of Adolescent Health,* 52(2), 280-286.

Jazaieri, H., Goldin, P., Werner, K., Ziv, M., Heimberg, R., Gross, J.J. (2012). A randomized clinical trial of mindfulness-based stress reduction versus aerobic exercise for social anxiety disorder. *Journal of Clinical Psychology,* 68:715-731.

Kerr, M. (March 29, 2012). *Elderly depression: Depression & aging.*

Accessed Feb. 5, 2015. Retrieved from http://www.healthline.com/health/depression/elderly-and-aging.

Kessler, R.C., Chiu, W.T., Demler, O., Walters, E.E. (2009). Prevalence, severity, and comorbidity of twelve-month DSM-IV disorders in the national comorbidity survey replication (NCS-R). *Archives of General Psychiatry*, 62(6), 617-27.

Kessler, R.C., et al. (2007). Lifetime prevalence and age-of-onset distributions of mental disorders in the World Health Organization's world mental health survey initiative. *World Psychiatry*, 6(3), 168-176.

Krans, B. (January 12, 2012). *How exercise can help bipolar disorder.* Accessed Jan. 3, 2015. Retrieved from http://www.healthline.com/health/bipolar-disorder/exercise#1

Kulas, M. (Jan. 28, 2015). *Social and emotional benefits of exercise.* Accessed Dec. 12, 2014. Retrieved from http://www.livestrong.com/article/477451-social-emotional-benefits-of-regular-exercise/

Kuper, S. (11 September 2009). *The Man Who Invented Exercise.* Financial Times. Accessed Sept. 12, 2014.

Lannem, A.M., Sørensen, M., Frøslie, K.F., & Hjeltnes, N. (2009). Incomplete spinal cord injury, exercise and life satisfaction. *Spinal Cord*, 47, 295–300.

Larson, E.B., Wang, L., Bowen, J.D., McCormick, W.C., Teri, L., Crane, P., & Kukull, W. (2006). Exercise is associated with reduced risk for incident dementia among persons 65 years of age and older. *Annals Of Internal Medicine*, 144(2), 73-81.

Latham, G.P. & Locke, E.A. (1991). Self-regulation through goal-setting. *Organizational Behavior and Human Decision Processes*, 50(2), 212-247.

Leith, L.M. (2009). *Foundations of exercise and mental health, 2nd ed.* Morgantown, WV: Fitness Information Technology.

Let's Move. (2015). *Make physical activity a part of your family's routine.* Accessed April 17, 2015. Retrieved from http://www.letsmove.gov/make-physical-activity-part-your-familys-routine

Let's Move. (2015). *Let's move health family calendar.* Accessed Aug. 9, 2015. Retrieved from http://www.letsmove.gov/sites/letsmove.gov/files/Family_Calendar.pdf

Lirgg, C. (1991). Gender differences in self-confidence in physical activity: A meta-analysis of recent studies. *Journal of Sport and Exercise Psychology*, 13, 294-310.

Locke, E.A. (1968). Toward a theory of task motivation and incentives. *Organizational Behavior and Human Performance*, 3(2), 157–189.

Locke, E.A., Shaw, K.N., Saari, L.M., & Latham, G.P. (1981). Goal setting and task performance: 1969–1980. *Psychological Bulletin*, 90(1), 125-152.

Lund, J. (2011). *For all eternity: practical tools for strengthening your marriage.* American Fork, UT: Covenant Communications.

Lunenburg, F.C. (2011). Goal-setting theory of motivation. *International Journal of Management, Business, and Administration*, (15)1, 1-6.

Mann, M., Hosman, C., Schaalma, H., & de Vries, N. (2004). Self-esteem in a broad-spectrum approach for mental health promotion. *Health Educ. Research*, 19(4), 357-372.

Markland, D. (2009). The mediating role of behavioural regulations in the relationship between perceived body size discrepancies and physical activity among adult women. *Hellenic Journal of Psychology*, 6, 169–182.

Gulati, M., Black, H., Shaw, L., Arnsdorf, M., Merz, N., Lauer, M, et al. (2005). The prognostic value of nomogram of exercise capacity in women. *New England Journal of Medicine*, 353(5), 468-75.

Mayo Clinic. (July 21, 2012). *Exercise and stress: Get moving to manage stress.* Accessed Jan. 5, 2015. Retrieved from http://www.mayoclinic .org/healthy-living/stress-management/in-depth/exercise-and-stress/ art-20044469?pg=1

Mayo Clinic. (Feb. 5, 2014). *Exercise: 7 benefits of regular physical activity.* Accessed Dec. 2, 2014. Retrieved from http://www.mayoclinic .org/healthy-living/fitness/in-depth/exercise/art-20048389?pg=1

Mental Health America. (n.d.) *Depression in older adults.* Accessed Feb. 5, 2015. Retrieved from http://www.mentalhealthamerica.net/ conditions/depression-older-adults#9

Mercola. (2014). *Sweating out sadness: How exercise can help the grieving process.* Accessed Feb. 7, 2015. Retrieved from http://fitness.mer cola.com/sites/fitness/archive/2014/06/27/exercise-grief.aspx

Mishler, A. (n.d.) *Yoga with Adrienne.* (YouTube channel.) Retrieved from https://www.youtube.com/channel/UCFKE7WVJfvaHW5q28 3SxchA?spfreload=10

Mohammed, T.A., Kucyi, A., Law, C.W., & McIntyre, R.S. (2009). Exercise and bipolar disorder: A review of neurobiological mediators. *Neruomol Med*, 11, 338-336.

Thomas Jefferson's Monticello. (n.d.). *Exercise.* Accessed September 14, 2015. Retrieved from https://www.monticello.org/site/research -and-collections/exercise

Moore, L.L., Lombardi, D.A., White, M.J., Campbell, S.A., Oliveria, S.A., Ellison, R.C. (1991). Influence of parents' physical activity levels on activity levels of young children. *Journal of Pediatrics*, 118, 215-219.

Morris, J.N., Crawford, M.D. (1958). Coronary heart disease and physical activity of work. *British Medical Journal*, 2(5111), 1485–1496.

Murray, C.J. & Lopez, A.D. (1997) Alternative projections of mortality and disability by cause 1990-2020: Global burden of disease study. *Lancet*, 349, 1498-1504.

Musick, M.A., Traphagan, J.W., Koenig, H.G., and Larsen, D.B. (2000). Spirituality in physical health and aging. *Journal of Adult Development*, 7(2).

National Alliance on Mental Illness. (2013). *Mental Illness Facts & Numbers*. Accessed February 2, 2015. http://www2.nami.org/fact sheets/mentalillness_factsheet.pdf

National Alliance on Mental Illness. (2014). *Depression in children and teens*. Accessed Jan. 17, 2015. Retrieved from http://www.nami.org/ Template.cfm?Section=By_Illness&template=/ContentManage ment/ContentDisplay.cfm&ContentID=88551

National Association for Sport and Physical Education. (1999). *The fitness equation: Physical activity + balanced diet = fit kids*. Reston, VA: National Association for Sport and Physical Education.

National Broadcasting Center News. (2004). *Global study finds mental illness widespread: Depression and anxiety often go untreated*. Accessed Jan. 10, 2015. Retrieved from http://www.nbcnews.com/ id/5111202/ns/health-mental_health/t/global-study-finds-mental-ill ness-widespread/#.VLf1HMaSVUQ

National Institute of Mental Health. (2008). *Introduction: mental health medications*. Accessed Jan. 7, 2015. Retrieved from http:// www.nimh.nih.gov/health/publications/mental-health-medications/ index.shtml

National Institute of Mental Health. (2009). *Treatment of children with mental illness*. Accessed May 22, 2015. Retrieved from http://www .nimh.nih.gov/health/publications/treatment-of-children-with-men tal-illness-fact-sheet/index.shtml

National Institute of Mental Health. (2015a). *Depression in children and adolescents: Fact sheet*. Accessed Jan. 17, 2015. Retrieved from http:// www.nimh.nih.gov/health/publications/depression-in-children-and -adolescents/index.html

National Institute of Mental Health. (2015b). *Major depression among adults*. Accessed Jan. 12, 2015. Retrieved from http://www.nimh .nih.gov/health/statistics/prevalence/major-depression-among -adults.shtml

National Institute of Mental Health. (2015c). *Women & depression: Discovering hope.* Accessed Jan. 20, 2015. Retrieved from http://www.nimh.nih.gov/health/publications/women-and-depression-discovering-hope/index.shtml

Nelson, M.E., Rejeski, W.J., Blair, S.N., et al. (2007). Physical activity and public health in older adults: Recommendation from the American College of Sports Medicine and the American Heart Association. *Circulation,* 116, 1094-1105.

North, T.C., McCullagh, E., & Tran, Z.V. (1990). Effects of exercise on depression. *Exercise and Sport Science Reviews, 18, 379-415.*

Northrup, C. (2006). *The wisdom of menopause (revised edition): Creating physical & emotional health during the change.* New York: Bantam Dell Publishing.

O'Connor, P.J., Raglin, J.S., & Martinsen, E.W. (2000) Physical activity, anxiety and anxiety disorders. *International Journal of Sports Psychology,* 31(2), 136-155.

Office of Disease Prevention and Health Promotion. (2008). *Physical activity guidelines for Americans.* Accessed Jan. 14, 2015. Retrieved from http://www.health.gov/paguidelines/pdf/paguide.pdf

Oliver, R. (1974). Expectancy theory predictions of salesmen's performance. *Journal of Marketing Research,* 11, 243-253.

Olderman, R. (2014). *15 easy ways to be healthier.* Accessed May 2, 2015. Retrieved from http://life.gaiam.com/article/15-easy-ways-be-healthier

Olson, S. (June 25, 2013). *Half of U.S. youth fails to meet physical activity standards: NIH calls for lifestyle changes.* Medical Daily. Accessed June 1, 2015. Retrieved from http://www.medicaldaily.com/half-us-youth-fails-meet-physical-activity-standards-nih-calls-lifestyle-changes-247133

Oppezzo, M. & Schwartz, D.L. (2014). Give your ideas some legs: The positive effect of walking on creative thinking. *Journal of Experimental Psychology: Learning, Memory, and Cognition,* 40(4), 1142-1152.

Orzech, K.M., Vivian, J., Torres, C.H., Armin, J., & Shaw, S.J. (2013). Diet and exercise adherence and practices among medically underserved patients with chronic disease: Variation across four ethnic groups. *Health Education Behavior,* 40(1), 56–66.

Otto, M.W. & Smits, J.A. (2011). *Exercise for mood and anxiety: Proven strategies for overcoming depression and enhancing well-being.* New York, NY: Oxford University Press.

Orzech, K.M., Vivian, J., Torres, C.H., Armin, J., & Shaw, S.J. (2013). Diet and exercise adherence and practices among medically underserved patients with chronic disease: variation across four ethnic groups. *Health Education & Behavior,* 40(1), 56-66.

Pagnin, D., de Queiroz, V., Stefano, P, & Cassaon, G. (2004). Efficacy of ECT in depression: a meta-analytic review. *The Journal of ECT,* 20(1), 13-20.

Palmer, J., Vacc, N., & Epstein, J. (1988). Adult inpatient alcoholics: physical exercise as a treatment intervention. *Psychosomatic Medicine,* 62(5), 633-638.

Pate, R.R. Pratt, M., Blair, S.N., Haskell, W.L., Macera, C.A., Bouchard, C., Buchner, D., Ettinger, W., et al. (1995). Physical activity and public health. *Journal of the American Medical Association,* 23, 402-407.

Pate, R.R., Baranowski, T., Dowda, M., Trost, S.G. (1996). Tracing of physical activity and physical fitness across the lifespan. *Medicine and Science of Sports and Exercise,* 28(1), 82-96.

Paulson, J.F., Bazemore, S.D. (2010). Prenatal and postpartum depression in fathers and its association with maternal depression: a meta-analysis. *JAMA,* 303(19).

Pavey, S. (2015). *Locke's goal-setting theory: Setting meaningful, challenging goals.* Accessed June 6, 2015. Retrieved from http://www.mindtools.com/pages/article/newHTE_87.html

Perou, R. et al. (2013). Mental health surveillance among children—United States, 2005-2011. *Center for Disease Control Morbidity and Mortality Weekly Report,* 62(02), 1-35.

Peterson, A. (2011). So cute, so hard on a marriage: After baby, men and women are unhappy in different ways; Pushing pre-emptive steps. *Wall Street Journal,* April 28.

PopSugar Fitness. (n..d.) PopSugar Fitness (YouTube channel). Accessed June 1, 2015. Retrieved from https://www.youtube.com/user/popsugartvfit

Postpartum Support International. *Depression during pregnancy and postpartum.* Accessed Jan. 14, 2015. Retrieved from http://postpartum.net/Get-the-Facts/Depression-During-Pregnancy-Postpartum.aspx

President's Council on Fitness, Sports, & Nutrition. (2015). *Facts and statistics, physical activity.* Accessed April 15, 2015. Retrieved from http://www.fitness.gov/resource-center/facts-and-statistics/

Prior, J. (1987). Conditioning exercise decreases premenstrual symptoms: A prospective controlled 6-month trial. *Fertility & Sterility,* 47(402).

Prochaska, J., Norcross, J., and Declemente, C. (2007). *Changing for good: A revolutionary six-stage program for overcoming bad habits and moving your life positively forward.* New York: HarperCollins.

Rader Programs. (2015). *Exercise therapy: Exercise does not have to be overly strenuous.* Accessed Jan. 2, 2015. Retrieved from http://www.raderprograms.com/treatment/exercise-therapy.html

Rainville, J., Hartigan, C., Martinez, E., Limke, J, Jouve, C., & Finno, M. (2004). Exercise as a treatment for chronic low back pain. *The Spine Journal,* 1(2), 106-115.

Ransdell, L.B., Eastep, E., Tayor, A., Oakland, D., Schmidt, J., Moyer-Mileur, L., & Shultz, B. (2003). Daughters and mothers exercising together (DAMET): Effects of home- and university-based interventions on physical activity behavior and family relations. *American Journal of Health Education,* 34(1).

Recovery.org. (2015). *What is exercise addiction?* Accessed Feb. 6, 2015. Retrieved from http://www.recovery.org/topics/exercise-addiction-recovery/

Recovery Ranch. (2015). *The effects of exercise on drug or alcohol rehab.* Accessed March 10, 2015. Retrieved from http://www.recoveryranch.com/articles/exercise-drug-alcohol-rehab/

Riggs, C.E. (1981). Endorphins, neurotransmitters and/or neuromodulators and exercise. In M.H. Sacks & M.L. Sachs (Eds.), *Psychology of Running* (pp. 224-230). Champaign, IL: Human Kinetics.

Rodriguez, D. (Feb. 14, 2011). Exercise, diet, and sleep: How they work together. In *Sleep in America,* 2012. Accessed Jan. 10, 2015. Retrieved from http://www.everydayhealth.com/health-report/healthy-sleep/exercise-diet-sleep.aspx

Rose, E., Larkin, D., Hands, B. Howard, B., Parker, H. (2009). Evidence for the validity of the children's attraction to physical activity (CAPA) questionnaire with young children. *Journal of Science Med Sport,* 12(5), 573-578.

Rosenbaum, S., Nguyen, D., Lenehan, T., Tiedemann, A., van der Ploeg, H., & Sherrington, C. (2011). Exercise augmentation compared to usual care for post traumatic stress disorder: a randomized controlled trial (the REAP study: Randomised Exercise Augmentation for PTSD), *BMC Psychiatry,* 11, 115.

Ryan, R. M., Deci, E. L. (2000). Self-determination theory and the facilitation of intrinsic motivation, social development, and well-being. *American psychologist,* 55(1), 68–78.

Ryan, R.M., Frederick, C.M., Lepes, D., Rubio, N., & Sheldoon, K.M. (1997). Intrinsic motivation and exercise adherence. *International Journal of Sports Psychology,* 28, 335-354.

Sasson, I. & Umberson, D.J. (2013). Widowhood and depression: New light on gender differences, selection, and psychological adjustment. *Journal of Gerontology, Psychology Sciences and Social Sciences*, series B, June 28.

Schmalz, D., Deane, G.D., Birch, L.L., & Davison, K.K. (2007). A longitudinal assessment of the links between physical activity and self-esteem in early adolescent non-Hispanic females. *Journal of Adolescent Health*, 41(6), 559-565.

Seabra, A.F., Mendonca, D.M., Goring, H.H., Thomis, M.A., Maia, J.A. (2008). Genetic and Environmental Factors in Familial Clustering in Physical Activity. *European Journal of Epidemiology*, 32(9), 1598-1600.

Seligman, M. (2004). *Authentic happiness: Utilizing the new positive psychology to realize your potential for lasting fulfillment*. New York: Atria Books.

Seligman, M. (2012). *Flourish: A visionary new understanding of happiness and wellbeing*. New York: Atria Books.

Sharma, A., Madaan, V., & Petty, F.D. (2006). Exercise for mental health. *Primary Care Companion Journal of Clinical Psychiatry*, 8(2), 106.

Shear, M.K. (2010). Complicated grief treatment: the theory, practice and outcomes. *Bereavement Care*, 29(3), 10–14.

Sichel, D. & Driscoll, J. (2000) *Women's moods: What every woman must know about hormones, the brain, and emotional health*. New York: HarperCollins.

Singh-Manoux, A., Hillsdon, M., Brunner, E., & Marmot, M., (2005) Effects of physical activity on cognitive functioning in middle age: Evidence from the Whitehall II Prospective Cohort Study. *American Journal of Public Health*, 95(12), 2252-58.

Smith, K. (2015). *Porn addiction statistics*. Accessed Jan. 12, 2015. Retrieved from http://www.guystuffcounseling.com/porn-addiction -statistics

Smith, P.J., Blumenthal, J.A., Hoffman, B.M., Cooper, H., Staruman, T.A., Welsh-Bohmer, K., Browndyke, J.N., & Sherwood, A. (2010). Aerobic exercise and neurocognitive performance: A meta-analytic review of randomized controlled trials. *Psychosomatic Medicine*, 72(3), 239-252.

Smits, J.A., Rosenfield, D., Powers, M.B., Behar, E., & Otto, M.W. (2008). Reducing anxiety sensitivity with exercise. *Depression and Anxiety*, 25, 689-699.

Sonstroem, R.J., Speliotis, E.D., & Fava, J.L. (1992). Perceived physical competence in adults: An examination of the physical self-perception profile. *Journal of Sport & Exercise Psychology*, 14(2), 207-221.

Substance Abuse and Mental Health Services Administration. (2015). *Alcohol, tobacco, & other drugs.* Accessed Sept. 4, 2015. Retrieved from http://www.samhsa.gov/atod

Substance Abuse and Mental Health Services Administration. (2014). Serious mental health challenges among older adolescents and young adults. *The CBHQ Report*, May 6.

Sung, I. (2013). Data points to behavioral health as a growing challenge for pediatricians. Accessed Jan. 14, 2015. Retrieved from http://www .athenahealth.com/blog/2013/10/28/data-points-to-behavioral -health-as-a-growing-challenge-for-pediatricians

Sussman, S., Lisha, N., & Griffiths, M. (2011). Prevalence of the addictions: A problem of the majority or the minority? *Eval. Health Prof.*, 34(1), 3-56.

Szabo, A. (2000). Physical activity and psychological well-being. In *Physical activity as a source of psychological dysfunction*, S. J. H. Biddle, K. R. Fox & S. H. Boutcher (Eds.). London: Routledge, pp. 130–195.

Taylor, C.B., Sallis, J.F., & Needle, R. (1985). The relation of physical activity and exercise to mental health. *Journal ListPublic Health Repv*, 100(2), Mar-Apr.

Teixeira, P.J, Carraca, V., Markland, D., Silva, M.N., & Ryan, R.M. (2008). Exercise, physical activity, and self-determination theory: a systematic review. *International Journal of Behavioral Nutrition and Physical Activity*, 9, 78.

Terman, M. & Terman, J.S. (2005). Light therapy for seasonal and non-seasonal depression: efficacy, protocol, safety, and side effects. *CNS Spectrum*, 10(8), 647-663.

Thayer, R. E. (2001) *Calm energy: How people regulate mood with food and exercise.* New York: Oxford University Press.

Thune, I., Brenn, T., Lund, E., & Gaard, M. (1997). Physical Activity and the Risk of Breast Cancer. *New England Journal of Medicine*, 1;336(18): 1269-75.

Thompson, J., & Blanton, P. (1987). Energy conservation and exercise dependence: a sympathetic arousal hypothesis. *Medicine & Science in Sports & Exercise*, 19(2), 91-99.

Torres, R. & Fernandez, F. (1995). Self-esteem and value of health as correlates of adolescent health behavior. *Adolescence*, 30(118), 403-12.

Trivedi, M.H. (2013). *The link between depression and physical symptoms.* Mental Illness Facts and Numbers. Accessed Jan. 3, 2015.

Retrieved from http://www2.nami.org/factsheets/mentalillness_fact sheet.pdf

Trost, S.G. & Loprinzi, P.D. (2011). Parental influences on physical Activity Behavior in children and adolescents: A brief review. *American Journal of Lifestyle Medicine*, 5(2), 171-181.

Trost, S.G., Owen, N., Bauman, A.E., Sallis, J.F., & Brown, W. (2002). Correlates of adults' participation in physical activity: review and update. *Medicine & Science in Sports & Exercise*, 34(12), 1996-2001.

University of Cambridge. (July 11, 2014). *Brain activity in sex addiction mirrors that of drug addiction.* Accessed June 1, 2015. Retrieved from http://www.cam.ac.uk/research/news/brain-activity-in-sex-addiction -mirrors-that-of-drug-addiction

U.S. Department of Agriculture. (2010). *Dietary guidelines for Americans, 2010.* Accessed Feb. 3, 2015. Retrieved from http://www.cnpp .usda.gov/dietaryguidelines.html

U.S. Department of Health and Human Services. (2008). *Physical activity guidelines for Americans.* Accessed Oct. 27, 2014. Retrieved from http://www.health.gov/PAGuidelines

U.S. Public Health Service. (2000). *Report of the Surgeon General's Conference on Children's Mental Health: A national action agenda.* Washington, DC: Department of Health and Human Services, 2000. Stock No. 017-024-01659-4 ISBN No. 0-16-050637-9.

University of Maryland Medical Center. (2013). *Stress.* Accessed Sept. 14, 2015. Retrieved from http://umm.edu/health/medical/reports/ articles/stress

University of Minnesota Duluth. (n.d.). *Personality and exercise.* Accessed September 12, 2015. Retrieved from http://www.d.umn .edu/—dmillsla/courses/Exercise%20Adherence/documents/Per sonalityExercise.pdf

Valliant, P.M. & Asu, M.E. (1985). Exercise and its effects on cognition and physiology in older adults. *Perceptual and Motor Skills*, 61, 1031-1038.

Van Grootheest, D.S., Beekman, A.T.F., Broese van Grouenou, M.I., and Deeg, D.J.H. (1999). Sex differences in depression after widowhood: Do men suffer more? *Soc Psychiatry Psychiatr Epidemiol*, 34, 391-398.

Volkow, N. (March 1, 2011). *Physical activity may prevent substance abuse.* National Institute on Drug Abuse. Accessed June 2, 2015. Retrieved from http://www.drugabuse.gov/news-events/nida-notes/ 2011/03/physical-activity-may-prevent-substance-abuse

Wellness Monthly. (Oct. 2012). *Moving through grief: Exercise can help*. Accessed Feb. 7, 2015. Retrieved from http://www.mansfield .edu/hr/upload/SEAP-October-2012.pdf

Whaley, D.E., & Schrider, A.F. (2005). The process of adult exercise adherence: Self-perceptions and competence. *The Sport Psychologist, 19*, 148–63.

Williams, M. A., Haskell, W. L., Ades, P. A., et al. (2007). Resistance exercise in individuals with and without cardiovascular disease: 2007 update: a scientific statement from the American Heart Association Council on Clinical Cardiology and Council on Nutrition, Physical Activity, and Metabolism. *Circulation*, 116, 572-84.

Wilson, K., & Brookfield, D. (2009). Effect of goal setting on motivation and adherence in a six-week exercise program. *International Journal of Sport and Exercise Physiology*, 6, 89–100.

Young, R. J. (1979). Effects of regular exercise on cognitive functioning and personality. *British Journal of Sports Medicine*, 13(3), 110-17.

Zhao, G., Ford, E.S., & Mokdad, A.H. (2008). Compliance with physical activity recommendations in US adults with diabetes. *Diabetic Medicine*, 25(2), 221-227.

Index

Note: Italicized page locators refer to figures.